EFFORTLESS
STYLE

EFFORTLESS STYLE

JUNE AMBROSE

WITH RICHARD BUSKIN
ILLUSTRATED BY AIMEE LEVY

SIMON SPOTLIGHT ENTERTAINMENT

NEW YORK   LONDON   TORONTO   SYDNEY

SSE

SIMON SPOTLIGHT ENTERTAINMENT

An imprint of Simon & Schuster

1230 Avenue of the Americas, New York, New York 10020

Text copyright © 2006 by June Ambrose

Illustrations copyright © 2006 by Aimee Levy

SIMON SPOTLIGHT ENTERTAINMENT and related logo are trademarks of Simon & Schuster, Inc.

Interior design by Joel Avirom and Jason Snyder

Manufactured in the United States of America

First Edition   10   9   8   7   6   5   4   3   2   1

Library of Congress Cataloging-in-Publication Data

Ambrose, June.

Effortless style / by June Ambrose with Richard Buskin ; illustrated by Aimee Levy.—1st ed.

p. cm.

ISBN-13: 978-1-4169-1896-7

ISBN-10: 1-4169-1896-5

[1. Clothing and dress. 2. Fashion.] I. Buskin, Richard. II. Title.

TT507.A643 2006

646'.3—dc22

2006010496

THIS BOOK IS DEDICATED TO MY LIFE PARTNERS,
MARC, CHANCE, AND SUMMER CHAMBLIN.
THANK YOU FOR INSPIRING ME!

ACKNOWLEDGMENTS

THIS book could not have been written without the love, support, and contributions of many.

Mommy, dearest, thank you for being the foundation and rock in my life. Your strength and commitment as a parent are indelible.

My sister, Wynell Jeffrey, and family, your love and support are a big part of my happiness.

My literary agent, Frank Weimann, thank you for holding my hand through this process.

Jen Bergstrom, thank you for caring enough about image and style to publish my book.

My editor, Patrick Price, and his secret weapon, Emily Westlake, thank you for having such a passion for fashion.

My book designer, Michael Nagin, your vision for this book super-exceeded my best expectations!

My celebrity clients, I thank you for giving me the creative outlet. Without you there would be no point of reference.

I would also like to gratefully acknowledge Phil Klein, Roger "Super-friends" McKenzie, my Modé Squad family (Orlee, Vincent, Brie, Sean, Becca), Oscar James, Ayinde Castro, Benny Medina, Andre Wright, Katherine Devendorf, Richard Buskin, Aimee Levy, Angelo Ellerbee, Marc Baptiste, Versace, Jean Paul Gaultier, Halston, Jacob & Co., Lorraine Schwartz, and Oscar de la Renta.

CONTENTS

EFFORTLESS
STYLE

INTRODUCTION

THERE
was a time, not too long ago, when celebrities dressed themselves. Actresses would grab a gown out of the closet or borrow one from the studio's wardrobe department and voilà, they were ready for the Oscars! These days, however, most stars won't even go to the grocery store without consulting their stylists first. And that's where I come in, hired not only to serve as a liaison between the designers and the celebs, pulling clothes for red carpet events, music videos, and photo shoots, but also to assemble a star's entire image.

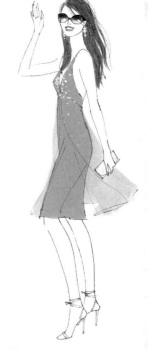

Today's fans expect their idols to always look hot, whether they're walking the dog or dolled up for the latest premiere. As a result, practically every item in celebrities' closets has been chosen by their stylists. We know their measurements, their likes, their dislikes, and what will keep their image hot and happening on a day-to-day basis. Yet although stars are virtually the only people who can afford to hire a stylist, that doesn't mean *you* aren't just as lost when trying to present yourself to the rest of the world.

I've worked with some of the biggest names in today's entertainment industry, but my message is that you don't need to *be* a star in order to look and feel like one. You just need some *star power*. And you'll get it by reading this book from cover to cover and learning how to make your wardrobe work for you within the confines of your body type and budget.

Women struggle every day with the question of image: "What will the boss think of me in this suit?" "Will my date fancy me if I wear this sweater?" And the age-old question that most people ask when they're debating whether to buy something: "Is this really *me?*"

Within these pages I will illustrate how the way you dress can have an impact on everything from your career goals to your overall mood. (That's right, a great ensemble can have the same effect as Prozac.) And once I've helped you find your own look and develop a style that will stand out from the crowd, you'll be able to exude the same effortless style as many of my clients, ranging from Mariah Carey, Sean "Puffy" Combs, Jay-Z, Missy Elliott, Will Smith, Mary J. Blige, and Jamie Foxx to Ashanti, Enrique Iglesias, Kelly Ripa, the Backstreet Boys, Macy Gray, and Kim Cattrall.

After a lifetime of wearing certain types of clothes and adhering to what you think looks good, all of this is going to be a reeducation process. Well, *take a chance*. That's what most celebrities do when they work with new stylists. And they take it in public. Well, if they can expose themselves on such a mass level, what do you have to lose? No one's going to be judging you like people are judging *them*. You're still going to have your job. They could possibly lose theirs. Just think about that if you're feeling a little apprehensive.

Great stars always know what they look good in and will never leave the house in something unbecoming. That doesn't mean they won't wear sweatpants and sneakers, but you can take it to the bank that those items will make a definite statement. As I tell my clients, they're the pioneers, they are forecasting the trends, and if they do it with confidence and conviction the marketplace is going to feed right into it. I mean, if they went in with disclaimers like, "Oh, you know, I'm not really sure how I feel about this outfit," their audience would automatically distrust them. Confidence and conviction are the key, so bear this in mind with whatever direction you choose to take as you progress through these chapters.

Normally, I assess my clients' characters and requirements after meeting them face-to-face. But since I can't do the same with you, it would be reasonable to wonder how I can impart my expertise and make it cater to your specific needs. Well, just think of me as your style architect. I'm going to give you the foundations that show how style is born, digging below the surface and building our way up by identifying your tastes, needs, and desires, and by providing thought-provoking ideas to help create your look. In the process, you'll be privy to the trade secrets that stylists use to translate fashion for their clients. And that is the magic right there. (You won't find it anywhere else.)

I want you to become emotionally attached to this book; to eventually understand and identify with the stars' thought processes. They exude what they exude because they think on a big scale. Playing dress-up is all about inspiration and emotion, and who you are should therefore be reflected in your garments. The ingredients are here within these pages. Put them together with my help and the results will be supertasty. Just remember: It won't happen overnight, and you might not get it from one read of this book. You may need to keep going over certain sections, all the time playing with clothes and accessories that will either bring you to the realization that you've reached your goal or that you're still working toward becoming that quintessential fashionista.

Whatever the scenario, rest assured, I *will* raise your fashion wattage. After all, life is a stage, we're all basically actors, and you can really change people's perceptions through the inherent power of *style*.

CHAPTER
ONE

DEFINING YOUR STYLE

WHEN

working with some of today's hottest stars, my mission is to interpret their style and transform it into an entire image. I find clothes that work for them, for their bodies, and for what they want to accomplish with their appearance, and the result is that many of the not-so-famous keep asking me, "How can I interpret what my *own* look should be?"

My response: "Just because you're not on the 'Billboard Hot 100' or making twenty million dollars per movie doesn't mean you can't have a style of your own; something memorable, something defined, something that will make people go, 'Wow, who *is* that?'"

This book is not just about how to find things that fit your body. It's also about how to truly define who you are and have your style—and other people's perceptions of you—reflect that. By defining who you are, you will have the star power to take risks and be more varied in terms of your style. Still, how do you achieve that star power? Well, with a little guidance it's possible to add some to both your life and your look, whether you're a lawyer, a legal secretary, a college student, or a housewife. So let's start with what you know.

Jot down the names of celebrities whose styles most impress you and could influence your own look. Do glamour girls like Sharon Stone, Jennifer Lopez, Beyoncé Knowles, and Catherine Zeta-Jones always strike you as impeccable? Or do funkier stars like Mary J. Blige and Gwen Stefani rev you up? Maybe you veer more toward the low-key bohemian, like Cameron Diaz or Jennifer Aniston. These people are all contemporary icons, yet you may also be influenced by those of the past, such as Jackie O, Ava Gardner, Dorothy Dandridge, or Marilyn Monroe.

On the current scene, one of my own favorites is Halle Berry, who has a very mod sense of style and is very slick. She wears simple clothes that really complement her figure without being overtly sexy. Because she's so pretty, she tones down the overt sexiness and plays more upon things that brush against the skin; bias-cut dresses, tight-fitting pencil skirts, or fitted trousers. She plays things up and down to offset her beauty. Then again, among my own clients I really admire Kelly Ripa— she's the type of girl who would prefer to be in jeans and a T-shirt, yet when she does have to get dressed up she's consistent in her look. It's a look of the moment, and she has many different moments, whether they're on the set or on the red carpet.

Still, regardless of your own preferences on the celebrity front, in the end it all comes down to the same thing—whoever your favorite fashion plates are, they probably have a look that has worked for them time and time again. And they, in turn, could help define the style that best works for you.

News flash: Most celebrities don't create a personal style all by themselves. Most have stylists who tell them what to wear, and you'll even see Grammy and Oscar winners thanking said stylists when they're pouring their hearts out at the podium. . . . Oh yeah, *they* know who really got them there!

That having been said, any good stylist is also aware of how important it is to give a girl a look that makes her feel confident and ready to take on all comers. After all, if you don't feel comfortable wearing certain garb, there's no point in concerning yourself over how expensive or fashionable it is. You'll simply look miserable. I mean, can you imagine

Mariah Carey dressing like Grace Kelly all the time? That would really make her itch, which would ultimately affect her performance. That's why I have absolutely no intention of turning you into some cookie-cutter Stepford wife. Instead, I want to help you embrace your *own* style, whatever that may be, and kick it into high gear.

One exercise I recommend is to rummage through your closet and pick a few outfits in which you feel especially confident. It could be that hot red camisole you wear with your favorite jeans and worn-in boots for all of your first dates. Or it could be that tailored suit in which you've aced every single job interview. Then again, how about that sexy pencil skirt together with the cashmere sweater that hugs your shape perfectly and makes you feel really sexy even on PMS days? The outfits that flatter you and make you feel strong are the ones that should form the basis for developing your own style. However, when trying to define your look, you must first determine your body type and then study your closet to find a *silhouette* that's common to your clothes.

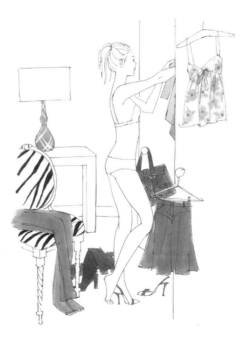

THE SILHOUETTE

This is the outline defined by your clothing, which might refer to an A-line garment that flares out from top to bottom; a bias-cut or knee-length dress; an off-the-shoulder or scoop-neck top; a V-neck versus a crew neck; a boot-cut versus a pencil-cut or slim-cut jean; or perhaps just long sleeves versus short sleeves. There are silhouettes that have been around for centuries, and we don't reinvent them.

Let's take a look in the mirror, remembering that it's just as important to zone in on our good points as on our assumed flaws. Do you have long legs or short legs? Are you hippy or curvy? And is this something that's ever going to change? You can't do much about your height, but you might intend to work on your shape. If not, it's about loving—or learning to love—who you are and working with that. This happens a lot with my celebrity clients. If they say, "I'm pear-shaped, I have no torso," we'll look at silhouettes that elongate their midsection, that cut right below their waist and create a waistline, giving them curve. It's all about working around the imperfection and learning to love what you have.

Don't think about the things you can't wear; think about what you *can* wear, because once you fall in love with the things that make you look exceptionally good, you'll start to think differently about yourself from the inside: "I don't care about my knock-knees, because no one knows about them aside from me. . . . And although I have broad hips, the man I love—or the guy who I hope loves me—is gonna love my hips too, because they won't change." Let your style help eliminate your insecurities.

Next, look at the favorite items in your wardrobe and see if they share a common silhouette. Do your favorite pants all happen to have long hems? If so, you probably feel at your best when you have an elongated leg. Are all of your tops a little on the snug side? Then you likely feel more sexy when you're showing a little boobage. Whether you feel more confident in jackets than in sweaters, short skirts rather than long skirts, or cap sleeves rather than sleeveless, the more you can identify what does and doesn't make you feel most comfortable and flatter your body, the better your wardrobe will work for you. What's more, it will also make future shopping trips a lot easier if you know that you never feel good in, say, pleated pants or boatneck tops. Unlike men, women are faced with so many options. To move ahead, it's critical to try to narrow things down.

Of course, you could say that if you're learning to love yourself, why put on a silhouette that accentuates only the body parts that work for you? Well, we all have a self-image with which we feel most comfortable. Some people are concerned about their bodies, others are more concerned about their lack of style. And whereas the former will pay attention to silhouettes, the latter's interest will be in the area of what colors and patterns to wear: "Can I wear stripes? Are stripes in? Is this pink lapel right for me?"

Many people don't necessarily care about a silhouette, what flatters them, or what they are *told* flatters them—it's all about what they feel confident wearing. That is why what you like is ultimately part of the solution to fixing your problem, whatever that problem might be. The key is to define who you are, what works for you, and how we can transform that into even more of a power statement.

If you work with what you already love, there are many ways to hone your personal effortless style. Say, for instance, that you really like the easy wearability of sweatshirts—what can we do to make them your own and make you superstylish? Can your body hold a belt around a particular sweatshirt? Can you put on a pair of tight jeans and heels with it? Or are you the kind of person who is completely miserable in a pair of heels? Maybe we can cut the crew neck off the sweatshirt and change it into a scoop neck, or remove the sleeves and wear it over a button-down shirt so that it becomes more fashion, less function. While you want to be daring, do bear in mind that when you're fresh out of the gate, you might make a mistake or two and ruin the odd garment. This is all part of trying and learning.

Now, if you don't even know what you like, let alone love, don't despair—*tons* of people with whom I work don't have a clue as to what they really like, yet when I help them discover things they can fall in love with, they develop dynamic new personalities. It's like that clichéd movie scene in which a dowdy secretary sheds her drab skirt and glasses, puts in contact lenses, lets her hair down, and squeezes into a figure-hugging top and tight jeans—suddenly, she's a total knockout. Well, you can achieve much the same result by using your wardrobe to define your attitude and express your unique personality.

What you shouldn't do is use it to *define* your personality. The personality should always come before the wardrobe. That is what some people miss. They believe the wardrobe comes first, and that's why the magic is missing. Without you, a garment is nothing. Clothes don't have a heartbeat. It's your *interpretation* that brings them alive. And whether you're dealing with bangles, a sports jacket, or sneakers, they can become part of your style. You can collect them, find different things that work really well with them, and then build around those items that have become a part of you.

WORK UP TO BEING BOLD WITH COLOR

People are so afraid of color, they normally choose only one at a time—no one thinks that pink can go with chocolate. And if they think that purple goes with yellow, that's probably just because the Lakers do. You have to understand tonality and what works well with your skin. So if, say, your basic black is going to be chocolate, establish a nice variety of chocolates, grays, blacks, and blues in your workable wardrobe. Never fill your wardrobe with just the one basic color. That's boring and makes you invisible. Instead, build your wardrobe with a subtle range of tones that work together, until you're more comfortable mixing in bolder hues and combinations like pink and brown, orange and powder blue.

THE STYLE SPECTRUM

It's important to distinguish whether you purchase clothes because they're trendy or to suit your lifestyle. People who are stylish regard what they buy as things they want to hold on to because they're a part of them, whereas trendies often shop for things because they're in fashion—they've seen them in magazines and they represent *now*. It's a case of choosing to value what's now or what's forever. However, style needn't be boxed in such strict categories. If your favorite piece of clothing went out of style ten years ago, that's fine—there will always be a way of updating it and making it *now*. Fashion evolves constantly, so don't get down if you're in love with that caftan and your body's changed since you bought it. If it's a great piece of fabric, let's put a belt around it. Or put some jewelry on it. *Reinvent* it.

✦ **TO GO FROM FRUMPY TO FOXY:** *Learn to play with your clothes. Those baggy sweatpants, for instance, can be salvaged by rolling down the waist, trading in the loose top for a tight T-shirt, and ditching the dirty white sneakers for some colorful Pumas. Then again, if you have a long peasant-style skirt, embellish it with a fitted top instead of a baggy shirt tied in a knot, replace the flip-flops with a little bit of heel, and add some long necklaces to elongate your torso area and make it really sexy. Likewise, you can put a belt around a frumpy sweater, wear a silky top underneath, and add tight leggings and a great pair of knee-high boots,* et voilà, c'est chic!

Those without a sense of style usually lean toward—or dive straight into—the no-nonsense simple or horribly overblown. The former tend to fall in love with one outfit or article of clothing and duplicate it in a variety of monochromatic colors. Imagine the female office executive who buys a parade of identical suits in black, brown, gray, and blue. No herringbones, plaids, or pinstripes; just clean, plain colors over a similar "assortment" of silk blouses. It's easy. And quickly boring. Style should never resemble a uniform. Meanwhile, at the other end of the spectrum, the overkill artists stare at magazine images with bulging eyes and just start blindly incorporating everything. In the process, they interpret what works for someone else, not for them.

You don't have to be obsessed with fashion to have a great sense of style. There's so much propaganda about what is in, what is out, what works, and what everyone should be wearing, as opposed to what simply feels right. In my case, having grown up and become a smarter shopper, I buy things that I know I'm going to look at ten or even fifteen years from now and think, "Okay, this still works for me." That's because they are classic, like a button-down shirt. There is *always* going to be a button-down shirt, just like there is always going to be a cashmere sweater, whether it's a cardigan, a turtleneck, a crew neck, whatever.

Establish what the basics are, and then you can get trendy with the accessories. Fashion is about the moment—it keeps moving and moving and moving—but style is forever. And if you're not a trend follower, don't dismiss fashion as a fickle hindrance. It's actually a help, because it encourages you to explore and to avoid the flat and the obvious. You should therefore consider adding patterns or embellishments to a plain piece. For instance, if you have a solid blouse that needs remixing, you could add an argyle sweater or a beaded cardigan for a little suave elegance. Just remember, things that are pearl-embellished make a better transition from day to evening than, say, a rhinestoned cardigan, which is definitely more attuned to evening wear.

♦ FOR A SEXY-GIRL LOOK: *Try throwing on a tight pair of embroidered stretch jeans with a low-cut caftan top, accentuating and showing off the lower part of your body. Or how about a denim jacket that you can make sleeveless? This really pairs well with fitted T-shirts and long, dressy skirts. Your jean jacket will keep things casual, while the accessories keep them chic.*

One of my clients recently told me she doesn't wear accessories. When I asked her why, she said, "Oh, it's too much work. I don't really know what I like."

"Well," I said, pointing to her ear stud, "*that's* an accessory."

She confessed that she liked small, simple things.

"Oh, that's interesting," I remarked. "Then let's start by looking at small, simple jewelry accessories."

From there it was about building on things that she didn't even think about, that were a part of her to begin with. You, too, may be in that position, unknowingly sporting accessories while being clueless as to how to take them to another level. Remember that simple but beautiful necklace your mom gave you when you were a teenager? How about layering it with the one somebody else gave you more recently? If you like the effect and experiment with more layering, who knows—you might end up with more of a gypsy look, become a little bohemian, and start to explore other cultures. This may sound completely out there, but if you're open-minded and willing to see where your experiments go, you could be in for a pleasant and interesting surprise.

✦ **FOR BOHEMIAN CHIC WITH AN ATHLETIC URBAN TWIST:** *The must-haves may include stylish tracksuits with crochet caps, baseball lids, matching sneakers, and driving loafers. This can translate from a younger lady to an older, more sophisticated woman—the former will play her athletic top with her embroidered stretch jeans, whereas the latter will find more power in the polished trousers, driving loafers, and cashmere zip-front hooded top.*

We are all so much less constricted by fashion dictates now than people were thirty or forty years ago. Today you can pretty much do what you want. Instead of an emphasis on silhouettes, designers are offering a refreshing array of textures and colors, and this gives even the fashion-conscious free rein to play around with ideas.

STYLISH ADVICE

One thing's for sure—I'm not the kind of person who says, "You've got a terrible sense of style." That's just an opinion, and I know the world is bigger than that. However, everyone can benefit from a little self-reflection. A lot of people dress the person they see in the mirror rather than the person they want to become. My advice is to leave your preconceptions at the front door.

When you deal with celebrities, they invariably know it all. And were I to take the direct route of telling people who think they have a great sense of style that they are wrong, it would only serve to end the conversation. Instead, I tactfully say something like, "I have a great suggestion for you: Because your personality is so big, because you have a beautiful smile and olive-colored skin, I would recommend that you wear *this* color and bring out those undertones. I mean, you have this amazing long neck and, oooh, you have *great breasts*, girl. Wear a V-neck so I can see more of *you*. And as for your legs and those gorgeous calves . . ."

That's the kind of problem solver I am, working with my clients' greatest attributes so that they stop thinking about being stylish and get that second skin going. Because once you've got that effortless second skin going, the silhouette that looks really good on your body along with the simple accessories, we can then set about giving you star power. So *let's get naked and start again!*

What do you love about yourself? Before you get dressed in the morning, how do you start your day? Do you put on your bra, panties, and a pair of heels before you apply your makeup? Or do you put on your bra and panties and just throw on your clothes? It's important for you to identify where your sexuality comes from, where you're most comfortable within yourself.

In my case, if I'm going to wear a tight pair of jeans, I have to put on a great bra because I'm sexy up top. You see, I'm short, so I love feeling tall, and that means I've got to put on my heels and my underwear before I start my day. On the other hand, some women love their bottom, so they put on a great pair of panties, nothing on top, along with their heels or their flats, and stand on their toes while they apply their lipstick and their eye shadow. That is what really helps them to start figuring out what clothes they're going to wear. And although I realize that, for most of you, your heels are the *last* things to go on before you rush out the door, you might just want to try wearing them as you select your outfit in order to feel a little taller and grander.

Of course, there are some women who hate everything about their bodies and they don't want to have to deal with them. If you count yourself among them, let's not deal with your body, let's just get dressed. What colors do you like? What kinds of fabric feel best on your skin? What is it about getting up in the morning and getting dressed that makes it easy for you? If there's a coat that you love, along with a certain dress, throw on the dress, throw on the coat, and then let's find something that excites you. *Let's have some fun.* We're going to accessorize—perhaps we'll find something great for the neck.

If you don't like your body, you're probably camouflaging it, detracting attention with a look that is likely based on hats or glasses and plenty of accessories. There's nothing wrong with opting to cover your body. In fact, if this is what makes you feel most attractive and comfortable, I encourage it . . . as long as you don't create a tent for yourself. You don't have to show your body to be happy and to feel beautiful.

✦ **TO GO FROM FOXY TO "FRUMPY":** *Take a high scoop-neck T-shirt and put on a pair of baggy jeans and UGG boots, and in an instant you'll be trendy-grungy. Or pay a visit to your boyfriend's or dad's closet, take a sweater that should naturally be oversize, and belt it over a fitted pair of jeans. The choice is yours.*

I believe in colors dictating your mood. You could put on green today, a bright, bright green like a chartreuse—a color that just makes you feel happy. Or if you're feeling really miserable, you can wear black—it's easy, it's monochromatic, you'll look decent and presentable, and you'll be able to set off about your business without having to think for the day. Then again, red may be your basic black, your blank canvas on which you start to create your second-skin color—it doesn't have to be black-black. It can be any color that serves the same purpose: red, gray, brown, you name it. Just make your basic black your own and use it as the foundation for your overall color chart.

✦ *It's hard to get it wrong when you're wearing black. The only time you can get it wrong is when you're wimpy and your black is ashy. In that case, one solution is to mix it with blue—the subtle contrast will be usable and sophisticated.*

A MATTER OF LIFESTYLE

Of course, one of the most important considerations is the lifestyle and needs toward which your wardrobe should be geared. Do you work in a corporate environment? Are you involved with the general public? Does socializing take up most of your days (and nights)? Or are you a stay-at-home mom whose appearance conforms to your own wishes rather than outside parameters? Then there's the little matter of whether you're a morning, day, or evening person.

Morning people jump out of bed right away without hitting the snooze button and have no problem starting their day without coffee. They need a really simple, clean wardrobe. Day people, who often pick up toward the afternoon, warrant more of a transitional wardrobe, containing things that can go from day to night. And night people, outgoing and social, often desire items with a little more inherent flair or drama. You could be one or more of these people. . . . If you're all three, you'll have a great wardrobe!

When I first meet my clients face-to-face, I look them over head to toe because that's who they really are, before having been influenced by my opinions or my expertise. That's who I want to see. It's like setting them free in a store and saying, "Pick something and come back," or putting a rack of clothes in their face and saying, "Pick something that you like that relates back to who you are."

I really think that sometimes, when people shop, they forget about who they are. They just buy stuff, yet they really should be thinking, "Who am *I*? What do *I* like?" Whereas some people like fitted jeans, others like baggy pants because they make them feel skinnier or make them feel boyish. The makeup of a woman's mind is very complicated. You're dealing with many factors, and it's difficult if you don't deal with these as separate parts.

During the course of this book, we'll be taking a look at your personality—whether you're carefree, at ease with your body, and like to just throw on some clothes; shy, self-conscious, and prefer to cover up; or tidy, fastidious, and like everything pressed. That, in conjunction with your silhouette and body type, as well as your preferred colors, textures, and patterns, will help determine what will work for you. Everything else—the accessories, ranging from the beads and bracelets, hats and necklaces, to the gloves and glasses, shoes and pocketbooks—is the gravy. It's the gravy and, ultimately, the attitude that give you the star power. Because if you don't make the people around you believe it, then neither will you.

All of which brings me back to my view of us as actors on the stage of life, able to change public perception and our own personae by way of the clothes we wear. I'm treating you the same way I treat the stars. And this isn't affected by the fact that celebs often have disposable incomes that most people can only dream about. After all, aside from the designer garb that they model on the red carpet, some are really into vintage, they have a great imagination, and they're open to taking a trip that is all about style.

These days, stores like H&M, Gap, Target, and Wal-Mart are selling premium-looking luxury-type goods, so again it's all about perception, style, and silhouette. Instead of spending thirty thousand dollars on a fur, you can get a great vintage fur coat and have it conditioned and relined for so much less. Nevertheless, some people aren't into vintage. Classic and iconic may work better for them, especially if they have a big personality and won't allow their clothing to upstage them. Effortless style is not about absolutes.

As we progress through this book, I want you to be on autopilot with regard to understanding the process of defining your own style. View it as a kind of freewheeling style-by-numbers formula, easy and nonintimidating, that lays down the foundation for the essential components of what is best for you. Just think of yourself as a blank canvas for the portrait you wish to create. You're drawing your own outline, determining who you are, and filling it in with the colors that you love, mixing them so that they work together.

When it comes to dressing celebrities, most of the looks that really get bashed in the press are the ones that are overconceptualized, overdone. Therefore, the trick that I'm employing within these pages is to avoid throwing a whole load of fashion at you. Instead, I'm going to give you the basics and then help you to build on top of that. First and foremost is your personality. This comes out in your clothing and your accessories. So take a good look at yourself, at your tastes, your needs, and your desires, and get ready to look and feel like a true celebrity!

And since deciding what looks best is often hard to do alone, it
really help to have an honest—and preferably *stylish*—friend who wi
act as your wardrobe consultant. (Share a bottle of wine—that always
brings out the truth.) If you don't feel comfortable wearing *anything* in
your closet, ask your consultant to help by giving certain outfits high
marks. If, on the other hand, you feel comfortable in *too many* things,
said consultant may well burst your little bubble. That's right; you might
be in far more need of style help than you ever realized.

CHAPTER
TWO

KNOW YOUR BODY, DRESS ACCORDINGLY

LET'S

get one thing straight: *Every* body type is perfect and manageable. We've been conditioned to think that a tall and skinny body is the only mannequin for fashion. However, the focus should be on universal style, as well as knowing and loving the body that you have to work with. Learning how to ingeniously put things together will transform you into your own fashion billboard.

The next truth is that not every single new trend is going to be flattering on you. I mean, if you have large breasts, high Empire-waist dresses are sure to make you look frumpy; if you're a little thick around the middle, you'd be best advised to stay well clear of cropped jackets, pleats, and anything that's too tight. Sheath-cut dresses are not a great idea if you're curvy; horizontal stripes or sailor pants won't be overly flattering if you're on the plump side; and if you're short, baby-doll dresses will make you look like a toddler.

The fact is, you can still look stylish even if a hot trend doesn't work for you. There's always more than one trend per season, so find ones that suit your shape and your tastes. And if you still can't find one that works for you, who cares? Trends go out of fashion just as fast as they come in, so you really won't be unhip for very long. Maybe a hint of a trend is the key. Instead of adopting an entire trendy ensemble, consider adding a small, trendy accessory as an accent. For instance, if you don't look good—or don't *think* you look good—in boho chic, you can buy a cool chunky necklace or a shrug and wear it with your usual preppy suit.

Looking good is way more important to my celebrity clients than merely being trendy, because they know how much better it is to wear things that flatter their bodies than things that are only going to be cool for the next few weeks.

Any trend should be done in moderation, so don't fill your wardrobe with the latest peasant shirts, tapered jeans, or fedoras. Take elements of each trend and slowly integrate them with your personal style. That way you won't be trapped into owning clothes for only one season. Well-dressed celebrities know they don't have to be the poster girls for every new trend that comes along, and you don't either. Your responsibility is to exaggerate who you are, bring out your fashionable alter ego, and convey an image that really speaks for you. Once you've figured it out, we'll cultivate your look so that it will remain timeless and enable you to dress it up or down for any occasion.

THE RIGHT UNDERWEAR

Dressing to feel sexier begins beneath your clothes. Underwear grants your body some form, control, and sensuality. And since underwear serves as the foundation for your second skin, it's important to get it right. That having been said, fancy undergarments are not always within everyone's price reach, so if you want to control your body's problem areas but can only afford basic items, these should probably include a good roll of gaffer tape—preferably with a husband or girlfriend helping you out with the application. Just start at the point where you want to pinch, and then wrap the tape as tightly as you can bear it. The illusion is cheap but effective. The only problem is, it won't last long on the dance floor. Gaffer tape is not an all-nighter. So if you can afford the expense, try some of the following less sticky solutions.

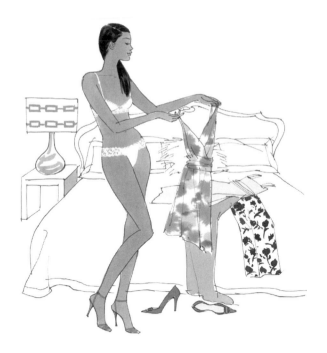

✦ If You Have a Small Chest

Go for a soft-boned Jezebel bustier. This has cups to give you a nice push-up and create a little bit more bust up top. It's very sexy. Then again, On Gossamer is also great if you have a very small bust, because it will seamlessly increase you by an entire cup size. It's like magic. I mean, you don't want to *look* like you're wearing a bustier bra—people will immediately know you're flat-chested. You want something that will give you what you need without it being obvious, and to that end, a cami that reaches to just below the rib cage can be both bust-enhancing and very stylish.

✦ If You Are Top-Heavy and Want to Minimize Your Chest

Olga makes attractive bras that are underwired and supersupportive, yet sexy, too. Just remember that improperly fitted bras can give the illusion of back fat, and wearing a tank slip top whose cups are too small will give you a boob deformity.

✦ IF YOU WANT TO SLIM DOWN YOUR MIDDLE AND KEEP IT SMOOTH ALL DAY

The Wacoal Hi-Cut brief works really well. It's extra high, with a heavy elastic waist that keeps the entire torso firm. And there's also the Nancy Ganz Belly Band brief, which is terrific for the woman who wants to slim down the thighs and smooth her kangaroo pouch. If you prefer a thong to a panty brief, you can go for the Flexees Control Thong by Maidenform. It cinches the tummy area and takes inches off your waist while also being comfortable. And for those of you who hate those nasty panty lines, there are Barely There briefs, which are so thin, they live up to their name.

✦ IF YOU WANT UNDERWEAR THAT WILL TRIM THE BUTT

Nancy Ganz and Maidenform Lycra shorts will always smooth out the bumps. They are perfect under slim-fitting pants, because they have lace edges that don't cause a line. And I also recommend the Spanx Mid-Thigh Bodysuit, which is similar to the liposuction body garment that patients are given following surgery. Very inconspicuous, it is the ultimate body glove. And for those of you who need control, the Spanx line offers other silhouettes to mask problem areas.

THE RIGHT CLOTHES, THE RIGHT ATTITUDE

Unless you're dressing a mannequin or someone on the runway, wearing the right clothes is not only about your body type but also about interpretation. It's about owning something and turning it into something that's you. It's about attitude. Just look at celebrities on the red carpet—they are exaggerated versions of style. You can derive energy just from watching their posture and the look in their eyes when they pose in a particular dress, and it's their sheer confidence that you really want to grab on to, because that confidence transforms you into a star. That's the power—*who* you become when you get decked out in your best outfit.

Okay, so you're not wearing a ten-thousand-dollar dress like your favorite star, but if your own outfit works for you, along with the hair, the makeup, and the earrings (faux diamonds work just as well as the real thing), you can spend an entire evening feeling like Raquel Welch. The confidence that you exude is the confidence of a star, from the way you stare to the way you hold your mouth. Stars don't put themselves on public display unless they're able to grab the attention of their audience, and that's the case even on their days off. At their frumpiest they are still starlike. The applause, the adulation, and their here-I-am attitude shape their style, their personalities, and how they carry themselves in their clothes.

Attitude is everything when you get dressed up. That's why, if a celebrity tries something and it feels forced and unnatural, we'll take it off and start again—they don't own it and they don't believe it. And if you don't believe it, you really shouldn't be wearing it. The goal is to wear something that feels comfortable and natural, something that will excite whoever you wish to turn on; fans, friends, future lovers, you name it.

Dressing according to your body type can be difficult to gauge. It's 99 percent about the fit. If, say, you want to buy a suit and you're bottom-heavy—perhaps a size ten at the bottom and a size six at the top—then you may become frustrated because you're looking for separates. Most women with that figure don't even *think* about buying a suit. However, there is a solution. Pay for alterations that will even out your body or wear more flattering silhouettes, with the right cut and solid, darker colors camouflaging your problem areas.

For more help, here are some other body-specific pointers.

✦ If You Have No Neck

I don't want to see you in a turtleneck or in a fur coat that's wrapped all the way up to your throat. You'll look like a floating head. Again, the goal is to even out your body, so stay with things that open you up, like heart-shaped necklines and V-necks, or deep scoop-neck

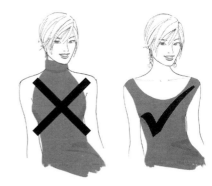

knits that will help to lengthen your neckline and broaden your shoulders. And if it's cold outside, you can do the same in layers, wearing a cashmere scarf to keep you warm. Unlike the turtleneck, you can always get rid of a scarf once indoors.

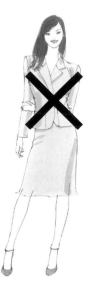

✦ IF YOU HAVE BROAD SHOULDERS

Try to avoid single-button jackets. They tend to pull and give you a Dallas Cowboys quarterback look. Two- and three-button jackets are much more flattering. When I worked with Kim Cattrall, she had a very athletic, muscular body, and finding a blazer to fit her was extremely difficult because her shoulders were quite broad and she had a high rib cage. So we went for off-the-shoulder tops, and she also looked really, really good in halter tops and things that accentuated her collarbone. Off-the-shoulder dresses are perfect for girls with broad shoulders.

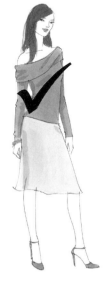

✦ IF YOU ARE PEAR-SHAPED

Stay away from pencil pants, slim leggings, and tank tops. Instead, go for A-line skirts; blouses and jackets that are less fitted and will even you out a little; and loose, side-fastening trousers whose lower waistband will halve the size of your butt. Just make sure you avoid trousers with on-seam slash pockets that are on the sides of the legs—these pucker out and add bulk to your hips. You'll be better off with smaller, flat-lying pockets that are positioned right above the hips. At the same time, keep well clear of the tent look—the oversize caftan that you may think hides all problems actually advertises them. When people get frustrated, the caftan is where they go to hide. Always try to silhouette and keep the shape of your body. It isn't horrifying to have curves and hips. In fact, it can be a really beautiful thing. You just want to highlight the bust to help even out your body.

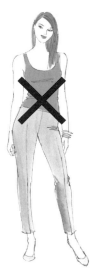

I recommend hip-length tailored cable-knit two- or three-button blazers to fill out sloping sho[ulders]. These separates can then be matched up with a sma[ll pair] of trousers or a straight skirt that doesn't narrow at the knees and intensify your hips. The pants should be dark—black, brown, chocolate, gray, navy—and pinstripes will also help to narrow the bottom. Just make sure the stripes are subtle and vertical, *not* horizontal! If, on the other hand, you have substantial thighs in addition to being bottom-heavy, a V-neck, chiffon-layered A-line dress with a high

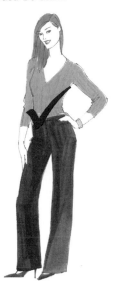

Empire waist will play down those problem areas below the rib cage. You'll retain shape while concealing the butt and thighs, and the chiffon layers will add sexiness to your look for that hot, star-studded moment.

✦ If You Have a Kangaroo Pouch

Tight outfits are a no-no. A gathered dress will create a distraction and hide the problem area. If it's in a solid matte color—nothing that has a sheen to it— it'll slim out the midsection and enable you to relax about the pouch. I normally use this strategy for my clients who are feeling a little chunky, and I also recommend coatdresses that will obscure the waistline.

✦ If You Have Long, Straight, Narrow Legs

It shouldn't come as a shock that you need to stay away from micro-miniskirts. You can look really amazing in high-waisted skirts that will give you more curve, boyish trousers that will provide bagginess in the areas where you lack meat, cropped or capri pants that will provide great proportion for your long pins, and cigarette pants that are just plain curvy and funky.

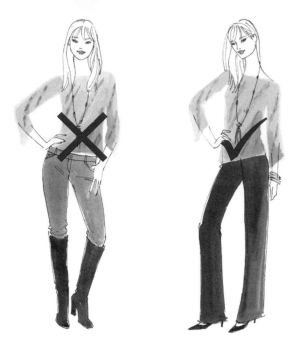

✦ If You Have Short Legs

I see it all the time, but tight jeans tucked into knee-high boots really don't work. All they do is leave you with about two inches of thigh and make your little legs look even shorter. That, my dear, is a *disaster*. Wear long, dark pants with heels to lengthen your lower body. Kick those knee-high boots to the curb, and stay away from the cropped pants that will take away whatever leg you have left.

✦ If You Have a Short Torso

Stay away from high-waisted skirts and trousers. The best things for you are tops that reach below the pelvis, similar-length blazers that silhouette the waist and lengthen your midsection, and Empire-waist dresses that are classic and will elongate your torso area . . . so long as they're not too wide. Likewise, tunics are stylish and brilliant over fitted jeans, but avoid wearing them as dresses unless you're in a music video.

You need to stay in heels and wear three-quarter jackets, not long trench coats. The jacket will camouflage some of the areas you are self-conscious about. This doesn't mean you can never take your jacket off. There are tops with sheer oversleeves, and amazing blousy bat-wing tops that are terrific for creating drama while concealing love handles and heavy arms. These should be paired with A-line or straight-cut skirts that don't cling to your hips but are just above the knees to give your legs added length, as well as slightly wide-legged trousers, fitted through the hips, that achieve the exact same thing. And, as you're now out of your shell, we might as well talk about other alternatives, such as the single-button blazer that plays up your top, creating a great waistline by way of a V from the neck down and an inverse V from the hem up to the button closure.

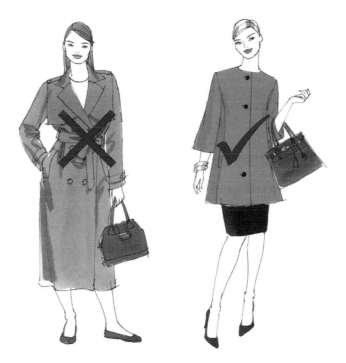

✦ If You Are Wafer Thin

There are people who have a complex about being too thin, but this problem is rarely addressed. If figure-hugging outfits are not for you, you can have a lot of fun with layers, such as pullovers with cardigans that are scaled to your size. Wearing things that are cut on the bias can also look really attractive, while A-line dresses will give you hips. What's more, stretchy tops with gathering at the bust, together with a brilliant push-up bra, will give the impression of cleavage that you never imagined existed. You can also get away with striped tops and sailor pants.

✦ If You Have the Perfect Model Figure

Congratulations, but don't get too cocky. Contrary to popular belief, you can't get away with anything from a designer dress to a potato sack (even if you do actually look great in both). There are, you see, things that no one should ever wear; the absolute no-no's, the don't-do's, the stay-away-from-at-all-costs. All of which leads us nicely into . . .

THE NO LIST

✦ Pantyhose with Open-Toed Shoes

I've seen too much of this, and now there's the even more ridiculous convention of wearing pantyhose with toe-capped shoes. Ugh!

✦ The Cowboy Boots and Cowboy Hat

However playful the concept might be, it's way too exaggerated when you put it all together. As with leopard print—a timeless must-have—the key is to not overdo it. When you overlive the moment, it turns cheesy. So don't do everything at once. Cowboy hats are campy and cute if you are on the beach, but they don't go with the boots if you're not on the ranch or living in the outback.

✦ Muumuus

They come, they go, they come, they go, but they are nothing more than granny housecoats or shapeless baby-doll dresses; a poor excuse for wanting to be comfortable and supposedly fashionable. Dreadful.

✦ Ponchos

These can be used as tablecloths, with flowers placed in the middle of the hole. They just cannot be manipulated to create a silhouette. Roomy they might be, but if you don't know how to use them they can prove disastrous. Some people who are top-heavy will throw them on to cover things up, but the result is that they end up looking like an end table, with little legs and no waist. Sweater pashmina throws are a much more classic and viable option.

✦ That Jacket from the 1980s You Really Need to Part With

Don't give me that line about things always coming back into fashion. They might evolve, but since their quality is often affected by mass production, they usually come back in a stronger, more sophisticated silhouette.

✦ Metallic Skirts and Trashy Open-Back Metallic Tops

Thanks to Bob Mackie and Britney Spears, teenage girls all over the world have wanted to wear these to school. Even some older women think it's okay to wear these monstrosities. However, unless you're performing in Vegas or appearing onstage in *La Cage aux Folles*, I wouldn't recommend that you incorporate this trend into your personal style.

✦ The Hooker

This plea for attention is so yesterday. As I tell every client, sexy is not about the garment, sexy is from within. I don't care what you do, there's no label on a miniskirt that says, "This will make you sexy." Some people confuse revealing with sexy. That's not what sexy is. I can psychologically help you identify it, but I can't purchase it for you. Of course, certain clothes can enhance sexiness, but it's all about how you wear it. If you don't feel sexy inside, it won't work.

PUTTING THE KNOWLEDGE INTO ACTION

Armed with the information in this chapter, you now know what looks good on your body. I think some window shopping may be in order. Of course, you can never really tell what something is like just by looking at it on the hanger, so if it appeals to you, *put it on*. And if you're an avid shopper, make friends out of your sales associates—they'll be honest with you when you ask for their opinions.

Your friendly and helpful sales associates should also help you shop for bargains in the store, because they know what's going on sale and when. Plus, when you're in the fitting room, it's much less stressful if you ask them to shop the store for some options to go with the pieces that you're trying on. They know the floor, so why tire yourself out looking for as many V-neck tops or heart-shaped necks or three-button jackets as they can find?

Once you have found your look and defined your style, you will realize how fashion translates so differently on a woman who naturally exudes sexy confidence versus one who is forced into a garment to find it. After all, if you wear a power suit but don't think like a commander-in-chief, you won't exude the desired energy. And that's because dressing the part won't do much to convince others that you haven't borrowed the suit. You must own the moment and become the total package. This all comes with self-assurance. Remember, if you know your body, you have the power.

CHAPTER THREE

WARDROBE ESSENTIALS

OKAY, so you don't need to buy into every trend that hits the runway, but there *are* certain items that every girl needs. Consider these your wardrobe foundation.

Essential pieces play well for anyone from a celebrity to a stay-at-home mom to that working woman who is constantly on the go. It's one thing to be going out in the evening and have time to really play with your outfit, but for the most part, we're talking about getting up and going. And in the majority of cases, whether your job is dealing with the kids, clients, the CEO, or the general public, you want to keep yourself looking good. To that end, you want something that's easy to throw on but still very chic, with which you can never go wrong. Avoid frustration by learning how to make your closet work for you.

Since few of us can afford whatever we want, what we're talking about here are the basics:

+ a pair of killer dark denims

+ a pair of rich-textured, neutral-colored trousers in khaki, black, brown, or gray

+ a silky white T-shirt, preferably fitted

- a V-neck, scoop-neck, turtleneck, or mock turtleneck sweater, whichever best complements your neckline

- a cardigan sweater with jewel embellishments or a detachable faux fur collar

- a tweed Chanel-like jacket, a crisp white button-down shirt—not your boyfriend's or husband's, but one that is fitted or fashionable, with darts in the waistline and exaggerated sleeves; something that screams opulence

- a neutral-colored cotton or cashmere jogging suit—so chic for travel

- a pencil or A-line skirt

- your Coco Chanel 1920s (or some other variation) little black dress

- the animal print overcoat that never goes out of style. Why? Because you're *not* pairing it with the matching hat, shoes, and gloves.

You can really work around ten or eleven pieces. Obviously, you'll need to rotate them, but at least if your closet burns down and you have to start all over again, this will be your *style survival kit*!

Of course, there are different strokes for different folks. Unless you're into the biker-girl look, a motorcycle jacket isn't an essential piece, and neither is a snakeskin python jacket—unless that's your thing. If you want to be a celebrity look-alike, you must own a real or faux fur coat. There's nothing more luxurious. You can build your essentials based on a particular look, while at the other end of the spectrum, shopaholics may consider *everything* to be essential. However, in general your wardrobe essentials should be timeless and multipurpose.

Whenever I take on new clients, I make sure they're well stocked with essentials that they can fall back on and feel good in. For instance, Kim Cattrall is a metropolitan diva, the kind of woman who transforms business casual into 100 percent glam. You can give her a great blazer with a stretchy pink tank top or camisole and a nice pair of jeans or a trumpet skirt, and she will naturally exude superstar power. Kim's athletic body and terrific arms mean that a sleeveless deep-V top goes a long way on her. It gives her length and sleekness. What's more, unlike certain other stars, she doesn't need major camouflage. She'll just give a great flip of the hair and twinkle of the eye and radiate sexiness via her collarbone and her neckline. If we could all be so lucky!

Now, I hope you don't think I'm saying that if you don't have a Kim Cattrall body, you will never look sexy in your clothes. What I *am* saying is that once you find those essential foundation pieces and the right frame of mind, they will enable your celebrity-style look to come to life. Here are some all-purpose essentials, capable of being combined with any number of items, that will find a place in most wardrobes.

YOUR FAVORITE JEANS

Jeans have become very expensive in the past few years, with the average price of a designer pair falling into the $150 range. Well, let me tell you, they're worth every penny. If you find a pair of jeans that are fashionable, fit you perfectly, and flatter your ass to no end, aren't they worth the price of admission?

Denim is definitely a second-skin essential. There is so much that evolves around it—just look at how a shirt or a pair of shoes can change the look of a pair of jeans. In terms of the fit, you can wear them loose and schleppy, you can wear them tight and skinny, and you can wear them casual-dressy with blazers and any kind of top. And then there are the different shades and washes that also play a role in the attitude of your denim pants: Distressed jeans are a lot more casual; dark jeans with a really clean finish and clean stitch can be worn day or night and look very professional; jeans with a lot of designs on them are more of a standout fashion piece. The same applies whenever you go into colors that are outside of traditional blue denim. If you're more of a straight arrow, a pair of, say, brown jeans may look dirty to you, whereas if you're a fashion risk taker, you'll maybe put a Burberry coat over them with a great button-down underneath and a cashmere sweater layer.

If you have at least three pair of jeans, you're good to go. You should own a pair to wear with heels, a weekend pair you can wreck—be they sandblast wash, antique, or simple faded—and a pair to wear with flats. This is your starter-kit jeans package. And if you are into denim and have a lifestyle and career that allow you to wear the fabric every day, I naturally encourage you to shop on. Make sure you buy a pair made of corduroy, a fun pair of denim capri pants, and a white pair of vintage wash. *Go for it*—this is a small price to pay for the most versatile second skin.

One of the best things about jeans is that they are seasonless. They can be worn all year round. What's more, jeans hold dirt well, they're very rugged, and they're everywhere. Walk onto a crowded street and there will be a sea of jeans. That's why there are so many brands. A whole load have come and gone, whereas the ones that have survived are those that are true to the fit. With denim, it's all about the fit. A

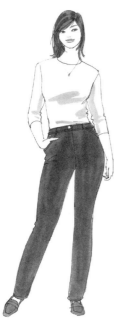

company can't be in the denim business if it doesn't come up with a fit that'll work for a girl who has a small waist and a big butt, or one who has a completely flat stomach and loves a low rise, or that girl who wants to wear boot-cut and high-waisted jeans without looking like a soccer mom.

There is one fit of jean that should be avoided at all costs: high-waisted jeans, with narrow bottoms. Producing a funnel, ice-cream-cone effect, these accentuate the difference between the ratios of the waist and hips, creating the illusion of broader hips and a wider butt. This sellout basically tells the world, "I've given up all hope of ever being sexy in jeans because I've had children."

If this is your attitude, then shame on you! Denims can be sophisticated and classic and easy . . . *if* you know how to shop for them. Look for
ones that have a good stretch—they will hold you in and (shock, horror)
even make you feel young and frisky. This kind of jean works really well
on full, curvy butts. If, on the other hand, your butt is sort of flat, I would
lean toward pocketless jeans that have a yoke. This style adds shape and
creates the illusion of more derriere. And then there are Tummy Tuck
jeans, which flatten your tummy, contour your hips, and lift your butt,
leaving you shapelier and sexier than jeans made for your daughter.

Boot-cut jeans, or those with a subtle flare leg, look
good on almost anyone. Fitted through the thigh and the
knee, they show the shape of the leg, and because the flare
balances the width of your thighs, they totally give you a
long, even shape. If you have excess fabric bunching up
between your crotch and thighs, this means you need a
shorter rise. All designers cut their low-rise jeans differently, some providing just enough to supplement a girl
who's used to wearing high-waisted jeans. And although
longer jeans give you longer legs, that doesn't mean you
should be stepping on the hems. Have the length altered,
and make sure they're a quarter of the way down your
heels so that you can also wear them with flats.

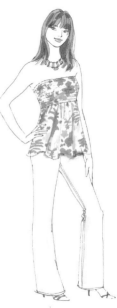

So, with all the different jeans out there, which ones
work best for you? Each brand has its own identifying look, but certain
popular brands really do work best for particular shapes.

Seven: These are really good if you have a larger bottom and need
some elasticity. Seven offers a range of different silhouettes, and what's
more, the jeans are now available in lower- and mid-priced stores.

Habitual: For the fashion-conscious girl with short legs. They'll hit
your back just above the waist and make you feel long, while their
smaller pockets will minimize your derriere.

Juicy Couture: These are great for the in-betweenie; the girl who's not too skinny but also not too plump.

AG: Perfect for the girl who has no hips or butt.

Joe's Jeans: Ideal for the girl who has major hips and butt.

Salt: These have a higher waist and are the best bet if you're looking for a longer rise and hate butt cleavage.

Jordache: These have great stretch and a silhouette that makes your legs look long. They work great with heels and boots. Jordache has been around forever, so moms know all about the brand, whereas their kids are just finding out.

Levi's 501: If you're more of an outdoorsy, tomboyish kind of girl, with a long torso and short legs, these jeans are made for you.

Bigger women sometimes need to have alterations to avoid that dragging crotch in the front due to their thighs rubbing together, and it *can* be difficult to find a jean that really works. However, no matter what your shape, jeans are never a bad idea. And even if you're large, the jeans should be as fitted as possible. Denim is a very thick fabric, and it can really hold you in, whereas if you wear it baggy it'll look sloppy. Just wear a longer top to cover your butt if you don't want it too clearly delineated—you're sure to look hip and cool. Find the ones that work for you by always trying on several pairs when you enter the fitting room. Never go in there with just one pair—that would be pointless, because they all fit differently, even if they're by the same designer and are labeled the same size. You can try jeans on for hours.

Once you find the right fit—one that you know is going to work for you even if the jeans stretch or shrink after being washed—you'll be able to wear that pair of pants every day and no one will notice. They'll swear it's a different pair. And if you need the legs to be shortened but want to keep the original detailing, have them hemmed the way the stars do by asking your tailor to alter and hem from the inside. It may cost a few dollars more, but again, it's worth it. Remember, if you want to maintain your dark-wash jeans, turn them inside out before you wash them. And dry-clean the pair that you can't afford to damage in any way.

✦ **MY JEANS PET PEEVE:** *the pair that's too tight at the waist. This results in the good old love handles and bubble that aren't really there, and all because you are convinced that your jeans are like leather shoes that just need to be broken in. "Oh, they'll stretch eventually." Yeah, right. That may be true for some parts of the jeans, but* never *the waist.*

THE LITTLE BLACK
(OR CHARCOAL GRAY) DRESS

Every girl needs one of these. Why? Because for all those occasions you're stuck agonizing over what to wear, be it a cocktail party, a funeral, a first date, or a job interview, you can rely on your little black or charcoal gray dress to carry you through with style. Both are such hard-contrast colors, the dress can be both stunning and slimming. And if you're already skinny, that's okay too. Just go for a fuller cut and a looser fabric. An A-line dress will give the illusion of curve, while a spandex dress will make you look like early Whitney Houston.

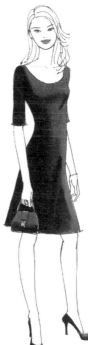

Black tends to fade, so invest in a dress and don't cheap out. In fact, if you need to spend a little more to get something in which you feel utterly invincible, like that *great* black dress made by Donna Karan, spend the extra bucks and don't feel guilty. Donna Karan is an all-American designer who definitely gets it. She's complicated in terms of her designs but simple in terms of the fit—she certainly knows how to drape a classic, timeless, silk jersey-knit dress that caters to all body types. And her pieces are always multifunctional. In the next chapter, I'll show you how to accessorize in such a way that your one black—or charcoal gray—dress can feel like five different outfits.

✦ *If you are conscious of your hips and want a little coverage while still looking stylish, try wearing a beautifully patterned car coat—an overcoat that ends at midthigh—over your little dress. That'll do the trick, while a herringbone or multicolored print will add just the right amount of pizzazz.*

THE RED DRESS

As an alternative to the black or charcoal gray dress, this is just as timeless, and if accessorized properly it can be worn day or night for almost any occasion. It's all about your personality, your complexion, and how extreme and severe you want to go with your classic dress. Black can be very severe on some women, almost making them austere and *too* mod. This is especially true if you have black hair. Indeed, if you have it in a bob and are wearing a black dress, you may look like an ice princess. And while that works for some women, others who want to be a bit more flirty might choose red as their basic color.

I wouldn't suggest that you wear a red satin dress during the day, but a red jersey-knit cotton dress can be worn both day and night. What's more, you can play down red with earth-tone colors by putting a beautiful camel-colored cardigan or a stone-colored jacket on top. Khaki plays things down really well in the springtime, and a darker tone such as chocolate does the same in the winter. Purple looks really beautiful with red too—this is a great transitional look in the fall. So start thinking beyond the basic black dress. Sure, black is timeless and it's also easy to put on, but it is just as easy to put on gray, red, brown, or navy.

THE WRAP DRESS

This is such a simple garment, it will work with practically any body type. Its silhouette provides loads of ways to manipulate your look, and should you need assistance smoothing out imperfections underneath, the most you'll have to do is wear the right body slimmer. This, in turn, will make you feel like a vixen and could very well provoke you into shortening your hemline. No wonder the wrap dress is a must-have—it'll save your life when you need to get glam in under five minutes.

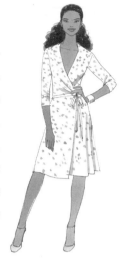

THE LONG GOWN

For a black-tie affair, a wedding, an engagement, a bar mitzvah, a night at the opera—this is essential evening wear. Some women just aren't able to cut it in a cocktail dress. They're either unhappy with their legs, or they feel that a cocktail dress makes them look cheap and like they're trying to be younger than they are. Then again, there are girls who feel a cocktail dress isn't dressy enough for certain occasions. In all cases, they'd prefer something long and elegant.

If you are a little large around the bottom, there are some beautiful A-line gowns, whereas a halter-neck gown is very flattering on a girl who has broad shoulders. Then again, a bustier girl should do strapless gowns, while someone who's conscious of back fat but has fallen for a gown that's low in the back should also try to fall in love with a cape or shawl that will cover the problem.

Once you've found a silhouette that works, a long gown will look fine regardless of your body type. It's like shopping for a wedding dress. Now you can start looking at the details. The cleaner and simpler the lines of the dress, the more you'll be able to add accessories and make it look different each time you wear it. Conversely, if you wear a really fancy-cut evening gown time and again, it's going to be highly recognized. So go for the cleaner silhouettes—the strapless or the halter-neck dresses that you can throw jackets or sweaters over. You can play with different things to make them seem new again every time you put them on: a different hairdo, different earrings, different gloves, whatever, depending on where you're going.

There are so many things you can do with a gown. You can remove spaghetti straps to make dresses strapless; you can add lace underneath to give the impression of a second layer; you can add a strap to a one-shoulder dress in order to give it a different dimension; you can cut it shorter and then add layers underneath to give the impression of a slip; you can cut it on the bias; you can add jewel embellishments to the shoulder straps; or you can add a back drape, which is a length of material attached either at the shoulder or the waist that flows over the area you want to hide. Be creative. And if you can't come up with ideas on your own, there's always the local tailor.

One more thing to consider is that the gown you own should be in a color that you love. Start by trying on a neutral color—gold, silver, champagne, black—and then go for that red dress, or burgundy if you think that will look better on you. You can even go with a dual tone. Just make sure you choose a color that you'll want to wear again and again—formal wear isn't cheap!

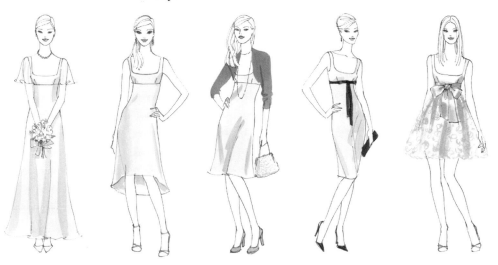

THE BLACK PANTS

These work well for any body type. It's just a matter of finding the right silhouette and trouser: pencil pants, cargos, gauchos, palazzos, capris, boot-cuts, knickers, you name it, in materials such as poplin, tulle, stretch wool, stretch cotton, or a poly-cotton blend. Black pants can be worn casual if you're just running out of the house, or smart, whether you're heading to a social event or the workplace.

From left to right: evening, casual, workplace

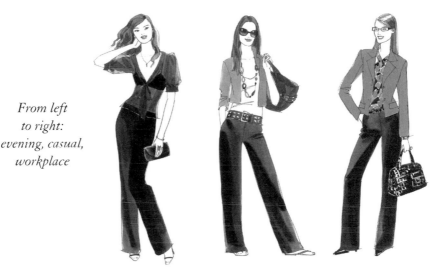

THE GRAY SKIRT

Be it A-line, midthigh, high-waisted, or pencil, this will work with any colors you want to match it up with. And you can wear it anywhere, whether it's a heavier wool or tweed in the winter, cotton or a more light-weight wool in the summer, or poplin all year round, with silk perfect for the evening. Another classic.

THE WHITE SHIRT

Regardless of your body type, keep it in your closet and you'll never go wrong. There is so much you can do with a white shirt, even a man's shirt. Putting on a man's shirt is really mod and beautiful. Every store carries this item and every designer has his or her own take on it, and you can wear it in *so* many ways—tucked in under a blazer for work, untucked over jeans for a crisp weekend look, or peeking out from under a sweater for a cute, preppy look.

Still, for effortless style you should also be properly accessorized, because your white shirt is more than just a bathrobe. It needs to be stark, powerful, and eye-awakening, so don't be afraid to do diamonds or pearls with it, or even a cool rock 'n' roll belt. And if you're going to tuck it under that blazer, make sure the blazer has plenty of color, whereas if it's worn over jeans it should accompany a great pair of high pumps. You can twist and tie your white shirt, belt it, or put a brooch on it. And even if you're into the preppy look, it should go with, say, a nice cardigan, a pearl accessory, and a driving cap. The white shirt shouldn't be flat. It needs to be exaggerated and have flair. And it also doesn't have to be a button-down with a regular collar, but perhaps have balloon sleeves with a ribbon finish on the neckline. The white shirt should look special.

THE BLACK TURTLENECK, THE BLACK V-NECK, THE BLACK TANK TOP, AND THE BLACK CAMISOLE

These tops have the same attributes as the white shirt. And if you're oversize, you can use any of these as a layer piece. With the black providing depth, a car coat will go fine over them, while underneath you'll be helped by the aforementioned body-slimming treatments.

THE PERFECT T-SHIRT

"A tee is just a tee," you say? Wrong. T-shirts can range from boxy and sloppy to tapered and truly sexy. So if you find a brand that fits you really well, showing off your shape instead of hiding it while still making you feel comfortable, buy in mass quantity! Get different colors so that you can wear your favorite tee all the time, and get even more if you want to always feel cute at the gym. James Perse, Theory, American Apparel, the Gap—all do amazing T-shirts at reasonable prices in a variety of sizes and colors. Wear them tight if you want to accentuate your shape, or loose if you prefer to underplay the bulges.

There are numerous things you can pair with a T-shirt to make it look cool or dress it up. Almost any kind of jacket will go with it, and if you're top-heavy and don't want to show off major cleavage, you can layer a T-shirt underneath a summer top—simply put a tight-fitting tank top underneath an A-line tank blouse, and that'll do the trick. A T-shirt can also be great with trousers, and you can even play it up with something like a beautiful, long, jeweled ballroom skirt. A simple tee will tone down a piece that is exaggerated and busy and place you between casual and fancy. That's the beauty of a T-shirt—it's so adaptable. Even in the wintertime, when it's not too cold and frosty, a tee can go with trousers, a fur coat, and some pearls. Now *that's* stylish.

THE TRENCH COAT

When the seasons change, you can wear layers underneath a trench coat for colder, damper days, or wear it as is on days that are a little nicer. The trench coat is always chic and glamorous. And we're talking about effortless style. Just look at Audrey Hepburn in *Breakfast at Tiffany's*. You can't go wrong. What's more, trench coats can serve as great cover-ups. A belted trench coat will give you a little more silhouette, while a Shaft leather jacket will just drown your body and make you look like you have no figure at all. The belted trench coat is very Sophia Loren. And it'll work really well with your button-down shirt, your tank top, or your turtleneck—it all depends on what superstar moment you want to create. A trench coat can be very mysterious, especially in conjunction with a fedora hat—just don't overdo things or you might look like you're in *The Pink Panther*.

THE PANTSUIT

Everyone should have a suit that has great color and texture and that can be worn in the office or at a dinner party. It should be considered your red-carpet suit (assuming that, for the average person, the red carpet is a hot night on the town). Stepping out the right way will make your evening a lot more memorable.

THE PASHMINA WRAP SWEATER

A sweater that is built like a pashmina, this has to be one of the best inventions. It is great for travel, business, and casual events, and it is pure genius. And it'll work perfectly with your short dress, your jeans, and even over your long gown, because you wear it short at the back and long at the front. In fact, a pashmina wrap will go with most of your essentials.

THE KILLER SWIMSUIT

Often, when women who are self-conscious about their bodies shop for bathing suits, they keep clear of the two-piece. However, that's just because they don't know the right silhouette to purchase. Even if you're small-chested, there are bathing suit tops that have structure to give you a lift and halter tops that will create cleavage that isn't there. At the same time, a low-cut bikini bottom that sits below your waistline will give you a longer torso area. Here are some different swimsuit scenarios.

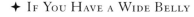

✦ If You Have a Wide Belly
The one-piece with gathering in the stomach area works really well. And if you want to create a waist where one doesn't exist, you can try on a bathing suit that has cutout sides that pull the eye in, or go with a belted suit.

✦ If You Want to Make Your Big Bottom Look the Best

Buy swimsuit separates that you can mix and match, with a smaller size up top and a larger size lower down. Some people think the boy short is a more modest way to go, but in truth the boy short doesn't really accommodate a full bottom. It makes the butt look bigger, whereas revealing a bit of the cheeks can also be flattering.

✦ If You Have a Boy-Shaped Body with a Tiny Butt and No Hips

Okay, now boy shorts *are* the answer.

✦ If You're Happy with a Sunburned Butt

Thong bikinis can be okay, although they're not very comfortable.

✦ If You Don't Worry About Support for Your Chest

Look to the ultimate adjustable bathing suit, the string bikini. You can cover fluctuations in weight by simply adjusting the string.

✦ If You Want to Minimize Your Hips

Try a V-bottom, where the side seams are above the hipbone and the center seam cuts about four inches below the belly button. It's a magical slimmer.

✦ If You Want Your Legs to Look Longer

Go for a high-cut swimsuit.

✦ If You Want to Downplay a Long Torso

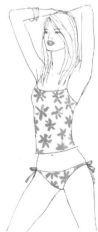

You can wear any two-piece, although you'll be better off with an off-the-shoulder two-piece swimsuit or a tankini. This is as opposed to a one-piece, which will exaggerate your long torso. A two-piece will create a visual break by showing a little skin.

✦ If You Have Love Handles

These will be accommodated by a string bikini. It sits low on the waist and you can adjust it, so there's no pinching.

✦ If You Have Larger Breasts

Opt for an athletic two-piece that will provide plenty of coverage and support, like a sports bra–style top.

✦ If You're Looking for an All-Over Body Slimmer

Chevron stripes running vertically all the way down are very flattering. Stay away from big prints that will pop out and make you look even bigger. Stick with small, sparser prints. And dark colors in a flat matte fabric will recede and make your figure appear smaller, while shiny fabrics are like a red flag for the sun and scream, "Look at all of my little bulges."

Check suits for inside construction. Make sure there are hidden features like underwiring, bra support, bust enhancers, double linings, and tummy trimmers. All of these panels will serve you well, so look for them when you're buying swimsuits . . . and look for Lycra content! A crochet bikini is good to pose in, but you don't want to get into the water with that kind of outfit.

Your wardrobe essentials comprise your workable wardrobe, and the pieces should all interact. It's like style by numbers—you know your closet works when each item that you have in it can match with everything else. Okay, so the trench coat won't go with the long dress, and the pashmina wrap should be kept apart from the A-line full skirt, but they're the exceptions.

Still, while your essentials should be partly based on personal taste, the brands that you decide to adopt as your second skin must also speak for your personality and what it could be. There are collections that really focus on a certain kind of look—with Ralph Lauren it's the town-

and-country, Aspen-meets-the-Hamptons type of look; while DKNY has a very New York City, young-but-professional vibe. Collections are all about the package, but you can also mix and match the elements. A conservative jacket can go really well with a tank top and a pair of jeans—it's a case of mixing two worlds, just like making an A-line skirt or wrap dress look more casual by adding a pair of boots. As long as all of the pieces are from the same season, you can play around.

Practice mixing and matching your wardrobe essentials, and try to incorporate what you already have. You'll be amazed by all the newly discovered options. And what's more, with the right accessories, you'll learn to use these essentials to create your own unique style.

CHAPTER FOUR
ACCESSORIZE LIKE A STAR

THE difference between dressing like a celeb and a non-celeb is in the details. Sure, it helps that a lot of the superstars' clothes are from Gucci or Pucci, but it also isn't hard to jazz up your H&M, Club Monaco, and J. Crew items so that you, too, stand out from the crowd.

No matter what style you're going for—preppy, funky, sexy, sophisticated, sporty—you can turn yourself into a more memorable dresser by adding some panache to everything you wear. There are the scarves, the gloves, the glasses, the hats, the jewelry, and a multitude of other accessories that will turn any ordinary outfit into a personal fashion statement. You are the one who sets the tone for your own look, and finding great accessories depends on your wardrobe and your taste. Remember, an accessory is supposed to enhance, not overwhelm, so do things in moderation and with a sense of style.

First, let's take a look at the must-have accessories, those multi-purpose essentials that should be in every girl's wardrobe. This amounts to quite a few goodies, so let's work our way from the top of your head to the tips of your fingers. (Shoes and bags require their own chapter. . . .)

✦ A Broad Fedora

This is masculine, yet it's also sexy and alluring, and it can be stiff or floppy depending on how mod you want to go. (More stiff = more mod.) Either way, this exaggerated version of the gangster hat is a very strong look, and as such it will definitely endow you with an air of mystery and danger. The fedora can be worn with a suit that boasts a beautiful loose pair of trousers and a sexy top underneath, as well as with belted over-coats. However, stay away from wearing your fedora with anything that has padded shoulders—you don't want to look like Dick Tracy. Everything else should be very soft and feminine. Alicia Keys is just one of many stars who live in a fedora. Also known as a trilby, this accessory was popular with women during the early 1950s, who wore it as a sporty hat, whereas today it is a sexy mode fashion crown!

✦ A Tam

Very Bonnie and Clyde, the tam-o'-shanter (a brimless, bobbled beret) is similar to the fedora in that it, too, has a little bit of man power. And

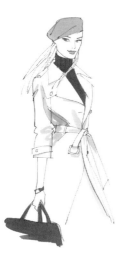

although it's mod, it isn't exaggerated, so you can blend it with other, bigger accessories that will definitely get noticed. Wear it with trench coats and turtlenecks—although you don't want to go Black Panther—and it will even play well with denim if you want to add some more energy. You can also wear your tam with an off-the-shoulder top or a ruffled shirt—anything that has a really noticeable collar. And what's more, it's a fashion perennial. After all, the beret has been worn by everyone from gangster's molls to prim-and-proper English schoolgirls!

✦ A Newsboy Cap

As sexy tomboy headwear, this looks great with jogging suits and denim, and is a playful way to make something that's really sporty a little more fashionable. Kind of like *Our Gang*.

✦ A Silk Scarf

This is a really beautiful accessory, whether it's worn loose and bonnetlike with big glasses, or tight as a head-band so that it's very mod and conveys more of a seventies

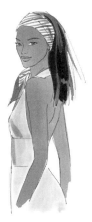

vibe. Wearing it tight is definitely more leisure oriented, because you'll probably have it on with a great sundress, and since a loose scarf is perfect for the chic woman on the go, you'll also need strong eyewear. The silk scarf is for the Foxy Brown kind of woman who has a really slick and slender face. When Gwen Stefani wears a scarf under her newsboy hat, she looks edgier and funkier. And while only certain people can pull that off, it's great layering headwear for the girl who is superstylish.

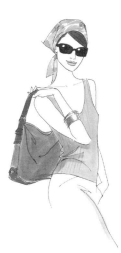

✦ A Fur Hat

This is drama, no matter how you bring it. Wear it big and watch people's heads turn. It looks great with cashmere coats and shearling, and it is very much Aspen ski meets the great metropolis. Sheer opulence.

✦ A Clip-on Hair Extension

Volume is the new genius accessory. Whether your hair is straight or curly, you can have your stylist work with different hairpieces to suit your tastes and needs. If you want more length, if you want more full-ness, these are must-haves. And if you've missed that hair appointment and have a last-minute dinner date or girls' night out at a club, you can just clip on your hairpiece and fly out the door. It's like hair on the go.

✦ Sunglasses

These are the biggest glam-accessories moment. Even in old Hollywood, if you put on eyewear and a big hat you were ready to go, whether you were lunching, sunning, or shopping. Glasses were an everyday thing. Now they represent exaggerated glamour, day or night. They have never gone out of style. Also, big glasses, together with really great hats, are essentials for stars who are always on the go, love accessories, and need a lot of high-fashion camouflage because their hair and makeup aren't always done. The hat and glasses make them feel more secure and complete their look. Take my word, they'll do the same for you.

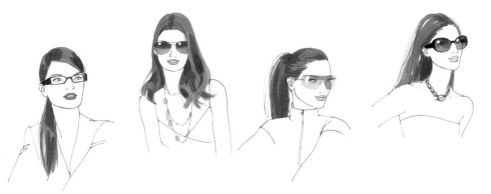

When it comes to superstar eyewear, not every girl can pull off the extra-large Jackie O look. It all depends on the shape and size of your face, as well as the style that suits *you*. For instance, if you want something more secretarial and serious, you may go for square, retro frames, whereas if you want something a little racier, then aviator-style frames may be the ones for you. If, on the other hand, you're a super-rock chick, you could look good in a wraparound frame. Whatever the story, I expect you to find a self-styled pair of dark glasses that fits the shape of your face and plays well with either a Saturday morning scarf or a fedora for a Monday head start.

Eyewear can set the tone for a look. So if you already wear glasses, I suggest that you have your prescription incorporated into your favorite pair of shades. Have fun with it. However, *please* be sure to have a lighter lens hue for the evening—there's nothing worse than a pair of Ray Charles glasses on a seeing fashionista.

THE EARS

Choose your upper accessories in moderation. If you wear a heavy earring, it should be viewed as the star on the Christmas tree, with all eyes drawn toward it. If your earring is small and dangling, or pressing against your ear, then it's an ornament that doesn't demand total attention.

✦ DIAMOND (OR FAUX DIAMOND) STUDS

Every girl should have them. They are, quite simply, an everyday classic. And you can wear clip-ons if your ears aren't pierced.

✦ PEARL (OR FAUX PEARL) STUDS

Understated and traditional, these are very, very big right now and they can go with anything. Again, clip-ons are optional, and just like the diamond studs, they suit any kind of headwear, while their proximity to the face allows you to wear chunkier jewelry around the neck. Some women enjoy collecting jewelry and wearing it in excess—it really becomes a part of them and their personal style. However, those who wear pearls are into simplicity, not excess.

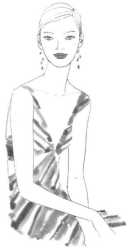

✦ LARGE ETHNIC OR CHANDELIER-STYLE EARRINGS

These are perfect when your hair is slick and pulled back. Mary J. Blige loves large, ornate, chandelier-style earrings. They work wonderfully with prints, be they paisley or floral, and some of the colored stones incorporated into ethnic earrings pick up the colors of the clothes really nicely. If you're going for more of a diamond chandelier, these scream evening and glamour, whereas you can take a blouse from day to evening simply by adding a large pair of precious-stone ethnic earrings. Just wear a more sparkly top with the ethnic earrings at night, and a more flat-textured top—maybe a cotton print—during the day. These accessories make a casual piece dressy and an evening piece with a diamond even more extraordinary.

✦ Hoop Earrings

These are a wonderful, very youthful-looking asset. When I work with celebrities, and something they're wearing feels too old and I want something more nondescript, a hoop earring never fails me. Whether it's a diamond hoop or simple silver or gold, it's the size that determines how the energy changes. The bigger you go, the more seventies the look becomes, whereas if you go smaller, the style is less conspicuous.

THE NECK

A woman's neck is the most beautiful thing. Collarbones are also very sexy. So you never want a pair of big earrings with a big necklace, because you only have so much neck to begin with, and it has to be a focal point.

You must pay attention to the length of your neck. If you have a long neck, wear something close to the throat, although I don't necessarily mean

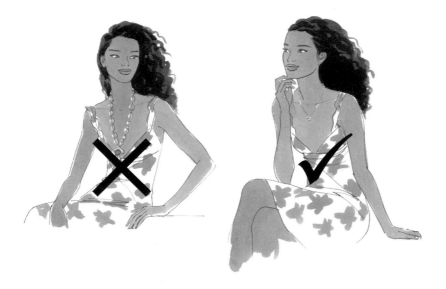

a choker. Chokers are more of a Victorian period piece that only work for really long and regal necks. They look very Gothic, and they never work during the day. So leave them in the past where they belong and go for a necklace that falls right below the collarbone. Things that lay on the collarbone are young, timeless, and elongating.

If you're going for a clean neckline, wear really big earrings. Pick the accessory with which you really want to be superaggressive and stick with that, because when you throw a whole bunch of accessories on top of yourself, you start to look like an accessory cart. You shouldn't be selling a product, you should be living it. Accessorizing is a very personal process. Take your time selecting pieces, collecting charm bracelets or pendants on chains, and put them together and play with them. That way, when you finally put them on they'll translate as something very unique to you.

✦ Layers

When you have a low, open-neck top, layered chains are really beautiful, creating something of a gypsy look. This is a very big trend that has recently evolved, and it looks like it's going to stay. Beforehand, you normally saw only certain types of women layering their jewelry, but now it's becoming the norm, and that has a lot to do with celebrity influence. Celebrities aren't afraid of exaggerating, overdoing, and overutilizing things that they have access to. However, I recommend that they only overdo one thing at a time.

✦ A Pearl Necklace

This classic says Oval Office. It's a very First Lady kind of look, and there's something very approachable about that, whereas when you go for chunky diamonds around the neck it's a more royal look. That's why Elizabeth Taylor loved the big diamonds—they were meant for Hollywood's royalty.

Of course, lots of stars use large necklaces to attract attention to their cleavage, but my advice to those offering a lot up top is to avoid throwing jewelry in between their boobs. Cleavage is an accessory in itself, and if you are showcasing yours in a low-cut dress, then that alone should be the focus for the evening. It's one or the other: the cleavage or the long jewelry. The two together are total overkill. If you must have something around your neck, go just below the collarbone and let it sit right above the chest. Keep it simple and small, otherwise you'll reduce the distance between your cleavage and your cheeks and you'll start to look shorter.

The necklace works best when set against a plain backdrop to showcase the jewelry. The neckline should either be open, showing plenty of flesh, or it should be really tight—simple and clean. Diamonds and other ornate precious stones will always take an ensemble from ordinary to extraordinary, but don't feel pressured to go to Harry Winston. Fabulous-looking jewelry can be purchased at stores that carry great fake accessories. After all, who wants to travel with an armed guard to the movies on a Friday night?

An icon like Oprah Winfrey can appear on her show wearing a cashmere twin set that's dripping in Fred Leighton ten-karat stones. Oprah's all about the luxury lifestyle. For centuries, diamonds have been the wealthy woman's accessory of choice, but even if you have cubic zirconia diamond copies, when paired with the right outfit they can go undetected.

✦ A FUR SCARF
While a man's thin necktie is a trendy item and completely optional, every girl should have a scarf to wrap or drape around her neck. Both functional and fashionable, it looks soft and beautiful.

✦ A PASHMINA SCARF
This versatile scarf can dress your outfits up or down. It looks great with sweaters and works really well as a transitional item when fall turns into winter, or when a summer's day becomes a chilly evening. You can wrap it in many different ways, and because it's inexpensive you can invest in more than one.

✦ A Gold Safety Pin

Use this on your scarf, to wrap a sweater, or just to keep something in place. If you utilize it for function, it's slick and simple enough to still be fashionable if someone catches a glimpse of your fastener, and it won't upstage your garment.

THE WAIST

✦ A Gold-Buckle Leather Belt

Timeless and classic, this is a celebrity staple, and it doesn't have to be made by Hermès. Just make sure the belt's color is neutral. Red and other bright colors are fine for fashion, but brown and black leather are your must-haves.

✦ A Broad Belt

This great accessory looks mod over a sweater . . . if you have a waist. However, if your torso is short and you have very little room to work with, stay away from it.

✦ A Skinny Belt

This *always* works with a great pair of trousers for any body type. And if you love the look of a belt over a sweater but don't have enough torso to do a broad belt, a thin belt is just as handsome.

✦ A Tie-on Belt

This simple sash works really well because you don't have to worry about size. It's so easy to manipulate that it can be worn on jeans, trousers, or a skirt—or over a blouse. In a fashion emergency, even a man's necktie will do the job if you need to hold your pants up. It's a really funky accessory.

THE ARMS, WRISTS, AND HANDS

There's plenty of style opportunity here, but again, don't overdo things. As a general rule, the busier your outfit is, the less jewelry you're going to need. The opposite also holds true. However, your pocketbook is another major hand accessory, so know when to stop. A dress may be a simple cut, but that doesn't mean it isn't a statement.

✦ BANGLES

Charm bracelets come and go, but these are forever. The more bangles you stack, the more bohemian-ethnic you appear, although this also depends on the outfit that you're wearing. Silver and gold bangles are more mod than bohemian, providing you with an elegant, effortless day look. If you're wearing a sleeveless top and your arms are bare, go for it. Don't pile them up to your elbows, but stack them to the point where they're still comfortable.

✦ A BRACELET

Silver, white gold, yellow gold, platinum—it's really down to what complements your skin tone. This is a must because it can play into *any* outfit.

✦ THE TRIO OF WATCHES

Since women and celebrities are on nobody's time but their own, for them a watch is more of a fashion statement. It's all about having one in silver, another in gold, and a very special one just for evenings.

✦ A BIG POCKETBOOK

Creating the impression that you have lots going on, a big pocketbook can serve as the focus of your simple-chic look. However, if you're less than five feet tall, I don't encourage you to throw a giant, knee-length bag over your shoulder. Leave that to tall girls or medium-height divas with a big personality.

✦ RINGS

The more ornate you go, the more your finger jewelry becomes a cocktail ring for the evening, whereas, say, a stacked ring can be worn both day and night. On the other hand (and forgive the pun), the oversize diamond ring is for the girl who is beyond glam and wants to make this very clear. The compromise is that you can't wear a great big stone and run around in cargo pants and sneakers . . . unless you're an Olsen twin.

EMBELLISHING YOUR CLOTHES

There are loads of ways to give added dimension to what you wear, but as with the aforementioned accessories, you can only go so far before you end up looking like a jumpsuited Elvis. Try new things but say no to excess.

✦ EMBROIDERY, RHINESTONES, STUDDING, BROOCHES

Choose one area of the garment to embellish and go for it. In fact, if you're into diamond embellishments such as brooches, try putting them on the strap of a really clean garment that needs very little enhancement. That's what I did with Mariah Carey, placing diamond brooches on the straps of her gown to give it a really glamorous edge. She dazzled everyone.

✦ DIAMANTES

Ooh, girl, I *love* that word. These are glittering, diamondlike stones that adorn clothes, textiles, and accessories. They're still very popular with Italian designers such as Dolce & Gabbana. Diamantes usually come in strips and are very easy to apply, so they're perfect on the waistband of jeans, or for making collars and sleeves more glamorous . . . so long as you use them in moderation.

✦ LACE

You can do accordion pleating, add it to the collar of a jacket, or use it to make a sleeve dickey or neck dickey. A trick that I employ all the time when a jacket sleeve is too short is to take an old sweater, cut the sleeves off, and make sleeve dickeys by pinning them inside the jacket sleeves. This gives the impression that you're layering when you're not, and no one realizes that the sleeve is too short.

DISTRESSING YOUR CLOTHES

Various methods are available to make new garments look more worn-in or vintage. Denim jeans are the most popular item to distress. But be careful, as distressing is not foolproof and could harm the garments. For example, people discovered that when they applied bleach to their jeans, the pants began to rot. Despite washing, the bleach never came out of the material, and the more they wore the jeans, the more they ripped, causing their intentional designer holes to mercilessly unravel. The solution now is to just apply coarse sandpaper to certain areas, again without overdoing it. Because if you distress something too much, it may truly stress *you* out.

FIND YOUR LOOK

There are so many trends that people brave when trying to come up with new looks. However, in order to make a real statement, it's important to actually find what your look is. And to do that, you can now mix and match your must-have accessories with your wardrobe essentials. It all depends on what you have and who you are. . . .

✦ IF YOU ARE A BOHEMIAN-ETHNIC TYPE
Great wood-beaded and stacked bangles may well be your passion. Still, don't overdo things by buying African print dashikis or draping yourself in Indian saris. When you get over the look, you'll be sorry that there's no flexibility in your wardrobe. Instead, just take the accessories from that look and tie them to the essential wardrobe pieces that we discussed in the last chapter. This will convey the right image while keeping you

more timeless and classic. A look like bohemian-ethnic chic plays well when introducing collector's items that you may have found at a second-hand shop or weekend flea market. You can also take vintage brooches and use them as pendants to be stacked with your thinner beaded chains, and beaded purses are another great ethnic element, found at Chinese markets and accessory bazaars. Jeweled slippers that you would normally buy to wear on an island vacation or European excursion can play well into your everyday wardrobe. Mixing this accessory with great skirts and trousers completes your leisure look.

✦ If You Are a Metropolitan Holly Golightly

Classic and mysterious, you probably drape yourself in black, and this plays really well with big glasses, gloves, and a tam. Your spring and winter gloves create the impression that you protect your hands and never get messy, and they also serve as great camouflage for a girl who's a couple of days past due for a manicure. Textured tights are de rigueur during the day (without looking Gothic). And the jewelry is simple: diamond studs or pearl earrings. The metropolitan Holly Golightly is the kind of girl who wears her hair really sleek and pulled back in a bun, while creating drama with a tam tilted to one side.

✦ If You're a Vixen Girl

There should be a pair of red pumps and plenty of baggy trousers in your closet, and you'll also have a lot of tight T-shirts with sweetheart necklines. For you, it's all about new sexy; it's all about silhouette and not necessarily your skin. People think that vixens are just about showing lots of cleavage and wearing miniskirts, but vixens are also not afraid of showing silhouettes of their bodies. Even if you are a full-figured woman, your skirts, pants, and trousers (perhaps a stretch pair with more of a boot-cut bottom) will all be super, super tight. A pair of austere glasses nicely offsets the overt sexiness.

✦ If You Want to Cultivate the Town-and-Country Look
Wear rain boots with your chino pants, as well as a neck scarf with your blazer. A woven leather or canvas bag works fine during leisure time, while on workdays you'll feel most comfortable wearing your estate jewelry pieces and textured alligator or tweed pumps.

✦ If You Are Into More of an Equestrian Look
Owning seven pairs of riding boots will come as no surprise to anyone, because that's your key accessory. However, riding caps are also great when you don't wear them with riding pants. Instead, the pants can look genius when matched with a great pair of pumps. Adding a white shirt and a broad belt will produce a great look, whereas introducing a riding cap to knee-high boots, a skirt, and a sweater vest is fine if you want to leave the gate and take off.

✦ If You Like the Preppy Look
Polo fitted tops with capris or fitted skirts may well be your thing. Accessorize these with kitten-heel shoes, pearls, and tennis bracelets, and don't forget your argyle socks!

✦ If You Want the Boy-Meets-Girl Look
You like to mix a lot of rough elements with soft and feminine items. The newsboy hat will blend with a trumpet skirt, while a silk blouse can go with a striped pair of gray trousers and platform shoes. Then again, how about wearing a broad belt with supercasual sweats? Or a trilby hat with supertight jeans?

✦ If You Are After the Victorian/Edwardian Look
Combine your maxi skirts with soft and moldable felt hats, dandy waistcoats, bold-stripe shirts, lots of texture, and belts that have antique buckles.

✦ If You're the Classic Punk
You're not afraid to cut your hair really, really edgy, such as in a Mohawk style. However, you'll also wear a beautiful oversize mohair sweater for

that deconstructed look, and indulge your classic side by mixing in something really slick, like a pair of Prada pants and even a cape to create quite a lot of drama. Add a patent leather belt and patent leather pumps or boots with some chunky jewelry and they will complete the effect. Just remember to use the patent leather in moderation. Cut-up fishnet stockings will create trashiness, but you can keep things classic by melding clean and classy garments with accessories that are inherently punk and edgy.

Accessories allow you to personalize your wardrobe and transform your look from conservative to classic, simple to sassy, anemic to endearing. Wearing an accessory that you love is like a strut down the catwalk. Nevertheless, while some women regard accessories as the foundation of their overall look, for others it's enough to pour their hearts and souls into garments that speak for themselves. In such cases, their outfits are the accessories.

So if finding the right accessories is just way too much trouble for you, don't feel pressured. It's all about evolving yourself and your look. There are plenty of stylish celebrities who don't accessorize all that much, either. Renée Zellweger, Kelly Ripa, Hilary Swank—none of these women are big on accessories. Their style is so sharp, they don't even need them. And the same goes for Angelina Jolie—her features are her accessories. She'll wear a pair of glasses, maybe a great Cartier watch, even a bangle or two, but that'll be it.

In your case, if you wear a dress with a really heavy print, that in itself is an accessory. So is a big ruffled top—you'll need nothing on your neck, and if it has exaggerated sleeves you'll definitely need nothing on your wrists. The cut as well as the pattern can therefore determine whether or not you need to accessorize. And if you do, then even your dog can serve as an accessory! It's about making the simpler things in your life more noticeable. Just remember, while bright, daring accessories in colors such as fuchsia, yellow, gold, or black can be your over-the-top statements for the season, please be careful to not take *too* long a walk on the wild side.

Your clothes, your tastes, your body silhouette—combined, these are the criteria for choosing the right accessories. And your age definitely plays a part too. While a younger girl often likes trinkets, chunkier jewelry tends to play well with the more sophisticated woman who has moved past her midthirties. That's not to say that you can't be funky and sassy and bold as you move up in years—personality plays a role as well. But, as you're about to see in the next chapter, it usually pays to wear things that don't regress or prematurely age you.

CHAPTER FIVE

DRESSING YOUR AGE

A COMMON

style mistake for women is to dress either too young or too old for their age. I mean, it's never a good idea for a gal in her fifties or sixties to wear pigtails and a baby-doll dress. However, much more often than that (but no less ridiculous) you find women in their twenties dressing like they're card-carrying members of AARP. Shapeless skirts at that matronly midcalf length; bland, ill-shaped jackets; baggy, high-waisted pants—if these are your fashion crimes, turn yourself in! Why on earth would you want to prematurely age yourself like that?

If you're equating "older" with "professional," there's a way to do it without making everyone think you've raided your grandma's closet. And remember, clothes express who you are, so don't even bother with that tired old line about it not mattering what you wear. It *does*. People are noticing and judging you every minute of the day, often to figure out who you are and if they want to get to know you. Well, the answer might lean toward "no" if you clearly can't put yourself together in the morning, or worse, can't even be bothered to try.

Effortless style evolves with the changes in your body and your lifestyle. When you're a carefree college girl, you look for more trendy and easy, comfortable pieces. Showing your curves is secondary. When you graduate and enter the workplace, you shop for clothing that is respectable and

. This can get lost in translation for some people who think ~~mpy~~ and conservative equals respect. The fact is, conservative is all ~~ntal~~—you can still be very proper with some color. Gone is the day of the solid blue button-down shirt because you're over thirty.

PROFESSIONAL POWER LOOKS

Even if you work in the stuffiest of offices, life can be brightened up by your look and your attitude. Never underestimate the power of color and texture. If your corporate uniform's comprised of navy blue, gray, and chocolate brown suits, that doesn't mean you can't punch them up with some color and patterns. Put shades of purple underneath the gray, turquoise to go with the chocolate, or a floral-print blouse under the navy blue. And if you want to be a little more sassy, go for a trumpet skirt instead of a pencil skirt, or trousers that are more fitted.

✦ If You Are a Young Power Broker

You don't need to grab attention with a scoop neck or stay safe with a superconservative high-neckline, straight dress that reaches just below the knee. Try wearing a flared skirt with movement and a slim-fitting jacket, or even a suit with a camisole if you're in a creative environment like an ad agency. You won't get away with a cami on Wall Street unless you layer it under your blouse and simply expose subtle hints of it. Just close your jacket according to how much you want to reveal and what is appropriate.

People in the corporate workplace get excited when a woman enters the office in a shirtdress or when she's wearing a pair of men's trousers and a vest. The look is very mod and strong and edgy, but it doesn't go too far. And it's also more than acceptable to add a strong belt to a very conservative dress and then throw a sweater over it.

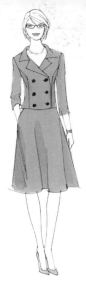

✦ If You Are an Older Power Broker

A two-piece suit is fine, but it's not an absolute necessity. I encourage separates, and a long jacket goes great with a narrow trouser. However, if you're going to add accessories, make sure they're daytime accessories and that you don't have a whole bunch of stuff on your wrist. Excessive amounts of bangles and bracelets are just not practical. A chunky necklace can really set the tone for your persona, as can a beautiful scarf and slinky pair of day gloves that you peel off as you walk through the office door . . . or as someone opens it for you.

DRESSING THROUGH THE DECADES

Okay, since I've already told you that your style can and should evolve as you grow older, here's a general age-related guide. Hardly all-encompassing to cover every taste and body type, but enough to illustrate the direction that should be taken as you roll through the years. If you're . . .

✦ In Your Late Teens

You probably prefer simple things like tank tops and T-shirts. They're easy. And when you want to be more fashionable and flirty but still classic, you can go for shorter items such as tennis skirts with polo shirts. In the winter, get creative by throwing your faux-fur bomber jacket on top of a suit or something dressier to achieve a kind of *Royal Tenenbaums* look: sporty mixed with luxury. That's sure to get you noticed.

✦ In Your Twenties

You still have your classic polo shirt, but your skirts are now a little bit longer. Mix that polo shirt with a pencil skirt or something fuller. In your teens you desired to make really bold statements and to separate yourself from the masses. Individuality was the objective, and you weren't afraid to take risks. People expected you to do crazy things. Many of those risks might still be on your agenda in your twenties, but you need to become a little more modest, especially if you have to consider the workplace.

This is the time to try a tight pair of jeans with a crisp, white button-down shirt, a bold and funky belt, and either a pair of boots or heels. If you don't feel so sure about your figure, go for solid colors and a very classic silhouette—not necessarily the tight jeans, but maybe a pair of black stretch pants or younger fitted trousers; not too tight, not too baggy.

EVENING WEAR FOR THE YOUNGER WOMAN

It's one thing trading on your youthful looks and vitality, but it's quite another being able to look both fresh *and* sophisticated when you slip into something special for an exclusive nighttime event. I live for a strapless dress on a young woman, as well as spaghetti straps and off-the-shoulder. Those simple lines always enable you to add cute little accessories. Even if you're top-heavy, they will minimize enough for you to throw a little sweater shrug on top—that way, you'll still see neckline without seeing cleavage. (Just stay away from the pashmina wraps and beaded brocade throws that are both aging and unnecessary.)

One thing designers have come to recognize is that a garment doesn't have to be long in order for it to be evening wear, and it really doesn't have to feel as debutante as it did before. You can add chunky jewelry to a very flirty young dress, whether it's floral print or a tube, or you can contrast an adult, sophisticated fabric like lace or heavy brocade with a silhouette that is really, really young, such as evening baby-doll dresses (if you're tall). This is a great way of mixing the two elements. At the same time, gloves are too costumey on a young girl, so stay away from them unless they are an intrinsic part of the look that you're trying to create.

✦ In Your Thirties

The twentysomething rules still apply. If your figure starts to head south, maybe after you've had a couple of kids, wear blousier but not baggy silhouettes. With extra curves you don't want to wear anything that is too tight or fabrics that are too thin. Go for monochromatic separates that will give you clean and classic lines that can never be ruined. You can even wear these underneath flattering pieces that have vertical detailing in terms of color, texture, and patterns.

✦ In Your Forties

There's a fair chance you now have that area of the tummy that you're very conscious of—the kangaroo pouch that just won't disappear. However, this can be redeemed by finding a great sports jacket. And, because you're in your forties, you'll match that single-breasted, one- to three-button jacket with either a pair of jeans or a pair of chinos and wear a crewneck top underneath. By now you should also be experimenting with hats and introducing more bold accessories into your life.

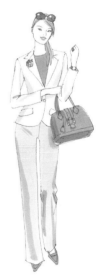

For those of you who feel like you're stylistically out of touch—perhaps you've been busy raising your family—just remember that you now have more time (and money) to shop and catch up. Buy great things that appeal to you, and stock up on versatile jackets, cardigans, and shirts. And forget "middle age" beginning at forty. These days, that takes place when you let it. Beforehand, don't shy away from dressing young*ish*. You may prefer a kitten heel to that four-inch stiletto, but it all depends on who you are.

✦ In Your Fifties

By now you know your body and should have settled into it. Still, you want to add a little drama to your life, so even though your bold pieces should still be very classic, your trench coat, for instance, might have a broader lapel or even an animal print if you're on the frisky, flamboyant side.

Quite rightly, most women of your age are not buying skins—they're not buying leather catsuits, they're not buying suede, because they either already own them or they simply think they're out of their lane. And they're not buying silk dresses that cling to their body. Instead, as the emphasis switches from sexy to sophisticated, they are much more into cotton and cashmere, as well as dresses that have beautiful lace embroidery and subtle beaded embellishments. Also, plain, satiny silk tops with a more casual trouser can still be very acceptable, giving you a hint of imagination. Mix sporty with dressy. Remember, fit and attitude play a big part. However, steer well clear of baggy pants up to the belly button. They are just wrong in so many ways.

Even if you still have the shape to go form-fitting, the textures of the pieces that you buy should be different—I don't want to see you in fitted, shiny, spandex leggings. Like a fine wine, your taste should age well, where your well-kept body is draped only in finer silks and durable fabrics with cleaner finishes, and you don't care for clothes that shift too much on the body, but prefer those that are naturally clingy where they need to be held.

Instead of showing cleavage, wear great body forms under boatneck tops, button-down shirts with the second button undone instead of the third, or lower scoop necks to expose collarbone and look more sexy. I love seeing an open neckline on a woman who is a little bit older. The result is more of a silhouetted body. Even at this age, you want to be noticed and complimented without being compromised, and things that give the illusion of a sixteen-year-old body under a well-draped garment will keep the male admirers wondering and wanting.

✦ In Your Sixties . . . and Beyond
Beforehand, this whole process was about evolving, but now you're done. This is your look. Yes, you might lose some weight and your body can still change, but even if you're Cher, there's only so much you can do. Accordingly, you'll often just build around the clothes that you already

have. You won't need to do as much shopping—unless you have a healthy disposable income—and that's why the pieces that you acquired in your forties and fifties are so important. They are the things that you fell in love with, so now try tying them back into your current wardrobe.

Some women pull out brooches that they had in their teens, along with vintage glasses and numerous other things that they've held on to. Well, it's okay to have separation anxiety. Just like some people don't want to leave the house they grew up in, some women feel the same way about clothing. You know, the "I've had this dress since I was in my thirties, and it still looks beautiful." That may well be true.

The practical woman who ages gracefully is usually a smarter shopper. She buys only what she really needs, as opposed to the young college girl who's burning up her new credit card. The older woman has her five classic belts, her silk scarves, and all of the other things that cost her a whole lot of money but are timeless. Even if she is going out to a black-tie event, she already has that dress.

With this in mind, go for silhouettes that are a little bit longer. They should be monochromatic or not too bright. Dual tones and very dark tones work much better. And they should also have great textures, like satin and silk, cashmere and wool, and the infamous knit jersey. At the same time, welcome more layers, but they should be *thin* layers—picture a car coat with loose-fitting trousers. You are working your way back toward easy.

THE THREE Ws

Of course, you might be one of those women who feels younger than you really are, and that's fine, but you don't ever want to be stuck in a sixteen-year-old state of mind. After all, a bold and brash young girl can afford to make mistakes and dress only for herself. That isn't your situation. As you grow older, you become more conscious of the Three Ws: the where, the when, and the why—*where* are you going, *when* are you going, *why* are you going—that guide style choices. You may have the energy of a sixteen-year-old, but the broad content of your adult day is vastly different from that of an adolescent, so your appearance should reflect that. Stay away from the hot pink Versace miniskirt and flip-flops when you're going to the office, and *please* don't try to turn heads in torn black stockings with Doc Martens combat boots.

If you want to keep men interested as you grow older, create a little mystery. When you're young, you can get away with revealing it all, but as the years go by those guys will have forgotten what it even looks like. As I always tell my clients, if you're going to show off your attributes, do it in moderation. And if you're working out but an area of your body is stubborn to change, simply accentuate your best parts. If, say, you like your calves, then go for calf-length skirts *as long as they have shape*; and if you prefer your forearm to the entire arm, go for jackets with elbow-length sleeves. Hide the negative, display the positive. You don't have to compromise your sense of style or who you are.

✦ *Some designers make versatile pieces for a wide range of customers. Theory, for instance, can work for a young girl as well as for an older woman. They have great boot-cut trousers that are classic, but because they are fitted and made with stretch material, they make the young girl feel good and comfortable while providing the older woman with the control that she needs—she can throw on a nice pair of chunky heels and feel like a stallion, whereas the younger person might wear wedges. It depends on what your age and body type can support.*

Once you hit middle age, there's no need to dress older than you are, such as wearing embroidered cardigan sets with "separates" that don't even detach, or frumpy one-piece outfits for women that should be reserved for those serving a prison sentence. It's all a case of mind over matter. Don't think old. Just look at the nice full-size collections of Dana Buchman and Elie Tahari. Designers are becoming a lot more clever as they realize that most older women don't want to feel that way, and the result is more fashion pieces with great colors and textures being added to their collections. These pieces are considered to be carry-over silhouettes—they take you over the bridge that spans the subtle body-changing age between your late twenties and midthirties when it's harder to lose weight, gravity kicks in, and—unless you're working out—your elasticity starts to go.

As discussed, your style naturally evolves with time. And as you gain more experience and confidence in terms of shopping, you will discover pieces in your wardrobe that continue to work for you during your evolution from young woman to more mature diva. Fashion, you see, is a revolving door. Over the decades, silhouettes have become less exaggerated—we haven't seen padded shoulders in years—but that doesn't mean garments have no structure. It simply means you don't have to wear football gear to score a touchdown!

STYLE ICONS, PAST AND PRESENT

The sleeker and less trend-driven you keep your silhouettes, the longer your garments will last. Effortless style is timeless. Let's look at some iconic role models whose natural sense of sophistication and Old Hollywood glamour continue to inspire us.

Take **Coco Chanel,** a sheer genius who aged gracefully. She knew what an accessory can do for a garment and was not afraid of excess in terms of her choices. She would throw on fifty strands of pearls with a big chunky cuff and a huge clip-on, and the result would look *just fabulous*.

Lena Horne, on the other hand, is an example of well-groomed elegance that is far less exaggerated than Coco. A forties- and fifties-style idol, Lena is a refined songstress who often wore a fishtail gown like a fashion goddess. And while retaining her physical beauty into old age, she has managed to always dress in a way that's stunning yet appropriate by way of simple drama: bell sleeves, regal glasses, and chic, short hair that accentuates her regal neck and strong jawline. Simple and uncomplicated, she has influenced artists such as Sade, Toni Braxton, Diahann Carroll, and Halle Berry. She is the epitome of natural beauty: never overstylized, yet iconic for decades.

And then there's **Audrey Hepburn**, always young at heart. Audrey had no qualms about pairing ballet slippers with a black jersey-knit dress, because she had an innocence that never died, even as she progressed past middle age. She truly was the epitome of her infamous screen character, Holly Golightly. Likewise, **Jackie Onassis**, the eternal debutante, still wore her satin gloves and string of pearls as she grew older. You can learn something from looking at all of these women. Nevertheless, not every girl is extremely chic. If your style is a little more laid-back, then you might want to take your lead from some of the contemporary stars.

Jane Fonda, now in her late sixties, continues to look great because she's very classic and metropolitan, and she knows the importance of a finished look. She's well aware of her physical attributes and is clearly confident in the woman she has become. She exudes strength, whether clean and casual in a white shirt and jeans or in a power suit. And she's also not afraid of color or putting on a great pair of fitted trousers.

Tina Turner is ravishing and inspirational to women in all age categories. The golden rule at her age is that miniskirts are to be stored away in time capsules. However, Ms. Tina keeps hope alive for the mature woman who still adores her great pair of legs. Of course, Tina's such a clever, timeless woman that she only wears her short skirts onstage, but her leisure days still find her in a tight pair of jeans, pointy-toed stilettos, and an off-the-shoulder sweater. She's forever bold and the chameleon of hip hair dresses.

A little lower down the age scale, those who get it right definitely include **Angela Bassett**. In her late forties, her strong, athletic body has really helped her realize that, as you go up in years, you're still in the mix.

She's conscious of how things naturally fit her body, and she doesn't overdo it. She's a style minimalist who doesn't take huge risks, just enough to be noticed.

Much the same can be said for English actress **Thandie Newton,** who, in her early thirties, can make wearing a simple tank top look like a silk blouse. Thandie can simplify a couture piece by way of tossed and slept-in hair, and completely convince you that this is the thing to do on an elegant night out. What's more, she is consistent. Even when pregnant and carrying a bump—a time when many women find it impossible to look effortlessly beautiful—she has displayed the power to blow off maternity wear and drive home the message that carrying the mother lode can be both stylish and stunning. With her beauty and grace, Thandie is the modern-day Lena Horne.

Lastly, you might want to observe **Reese Witherspoon.** She has that Southern belle kind of look, but she knows what is appropriate when she's in her working mom mode and is unafraid of throwing on jeans, her sweater, and a backpack. Then, when it's time to be a movie star, she's the sweetest and best put-together thing in Tinseltown. She'll wear a circle skirt with a tank top and a cardigan, and look just perfect for a gal in her late twenties.

Regardless of your age, if you want to accentuate a part of your figure, don't be overt. Pick one attribute and reveal only that for the night. For instance . . .

✦ If the Nape of Your Neck Is Very Strong

Wear something with a low back and high front. Don't show cleavage at the front *and* cleavage at the back. And I also don't want to see butt cleavage. Just feature the nape of your neck as well as your arms.

BORROWING INSTEAD OF BUYING

You either own it or you don't, so if you do want to try something as a one-off, it makes sense to borrow rather than buy. (This is a concept that all celebrities are familiar with!) Otherwise, making that investment will be so hard and, in all likelihood, pointless, because you won't live in the outfit and will probably never wear it again. There are companies catering to this—you can even rent a purse or pocketbook from places like Bag, Borrow or Steal and feel like Cinderella for the night! In fact, if it's going to be a Cinderella event—something very, very grand that will garner you a lot of attention—then you'll need something memorable for such a memorable evening, and in that case, unless you already have the perfect outfit, it might be worth borrowing, rather than buying something extravagant that will remain forever untouched in your closet afterward.

Here are just a few great rental places:

Bag, Borrow or Steal
Tel: (866) 922-2267
www.bagborroworsteal.com

Allan and Suzi
416 Amsterdam Avenue
New York, NY 10024
Tel: (212) 724-7445
www.allanandsuzi.net

Myrjan
235 St. Marks Avenue
Brooklyn, NY 11238
Tel: (718) 623-3848
www.myrjan.com

Alexandria's Formal Gown
Rental
112 Main Street
Roseville, California 95678
Tel: (916) 787-0900
www.alexandriasformal.com

One Night Stand
8 Chelsea Manor Studios
Flood Street
London SW3 5SR, England
Tel: +44-(0)20-7352-4848
www.onenightstand.co.uk

And if you want to save money by purchasing a high-end designer look-alike, Jovani Fashions creates everything from prom to mother-of-the-bride and red-carpet-for-less: www.jovani.com.

✦ If You Want to Show Off Your Legs

Pick something with a really high split, not to the hipbone but to midthigh. At that point, it's okay for you to show shoulder, collarbone, and a little bit of cleavage, but not too much.

✦ If You're Going for Deep Cleavage

Wear something knee-length. Believe me, it'll look very, very supersexy. Do *not* go cleavage and miniskirt . . . unless you're pole-dancing or standing on the street corner. I don't think you should sell it all at one time.

✦ If You Want to Flaunt Your Curvy Derriere

You also should have a slim waist. A hugging skirt will place all the focus firmly on the butt area. Jennifer Lopez gets away with it all the time. Then again, if you're pear-shaped, an A-line, flirty-colored halter-neck dress would be equally flattering.

I think it's very important to understand that, while you do have to alter your fit and sizes to accommodate your ever-changing body, and be conscious of what's acceptable for you at this stage in your life, you *don't* have to compromise your personal style because of age. As people grow older, they become afraid of losing their sense of style due to all the physical changes. However, never abandon your will for being creative or your ability to interpret fashion.

I hope that, by reading this book, we're starting to connect and build a relationship, and that this in turn will reassure you that there is a spark in everyone and that stars never dwindle.

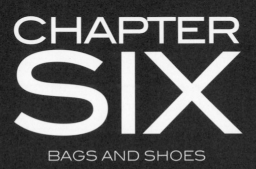

CHAPTER
SIX

BAGS AND SHOES

SOME

things really aren't worth the money. Trendy pieces, for the most part, fall into this category unless you have Paris Hilton's bank account. After all, why pay four hundred dollars for a poncho that's only going to be in style for a month? If you *are* going to spend your money on something, go for those items that are guaranteed to provide the biggest bang for the buck: shoes and bags.

BAGS

It doesn't matter if you're wearing Old Navy jeans and a Gap sweater—if you have a Louis Vuitton bag on your arm and Gucci loafers on your feet, you'll look and feel like a star. Before shuddering at the thought of going into debt for a designer label, consider several reasons why you should spend freely on a classic bag:

+ If you take good care of it, it will last forever.

+ If you buy it in a neutral color, you can wear it with everything, every season, for years to come.

+ You will carry yourself with confidence while clutching that special bag.

The one drawback to purchasing a classic is the cost. Most people are not comfortable with spending what can amount to a thousand dollars or more on an accessory. However, you should think of it as an investment. Say you drop $895 on a beautiful Marc Jacobs multipocket leather bag that you've been eyeing for the longest time. If you wear it every day for the next two years, that's only $1.22 a day—less than the price of a cup of coffee or a subway ride!

Now, if you're still not on board, or if that kind of expense is simply out of your price range, you could always consider purchasing a fake. Yep, I've said it—if you can get your hands on a good (and I mean *good*) faux Chanel, Gucci, or Louis Vuitton, and you carry yourself like it's real with your head held high) you'll probably get away with it. Sure, a few people will be able to tell the difference, but if you accessorize like a star and have the right attitude, most folks will be none the wiser.

The fact is, certain widely recognized designer bags are assumed to be fakes. Bold and iconic, they are constantly knocked off, and this has grown to the point where, from most people's point of view, it's impossible to tell if the bag is authentic. Now, I'm not endorsing the fraudsters or disparaging the real thing—quality is quality, no matter what, and the goal here is to look and feel like a true celeb. But if funds are limited, you may want to think about how to invest your money. Do you really want to spend three thousand dollars on a purse that many people will assume to be fake? Or will the look-alike with the similar logo achieve the desired effect for far less cash?

✦ MUST-HAVE BAGS

Like an antique Christmas ornament, the right bag may not be the star atop the tree, but you can certainly admire it from afar. Even if there's nothing else that you like about a person's outfit, if they're carrying a killer purse you can still say, "Great bag!" Carry one yourself and bask in the compliments that'll come your way. Nevertheless, while some bags can be worn with practically any outfit, you sometimes need to choose your accessories based on function and, more important, your personality. Your income will help determine how many bags you're able to acquire, but your lifestyle should be taken into consideration first. So review the options listed below and, if you're able to afford it, decide which bag suits you best for each occasion.

The Handbag

Not meant to be worn on your shoulder but on your forearm and wrist, this is a ladylike bag because it forces you to carry it in a certain dainty way and inspires you to display feminine mannerisms. If your taste is girly, splurge on one fabulous handbag that reflects your personality and you'll end up taking it everywhere.

The Tote Bag

Handbags come in many shapes and sizes, but they probably won't work if you want to carry around a lot of paperwork. A soft and open tote bag would be best. So if you're the kind of girl who wants to carry her cosmetics, her cell phone, her camera, and her sneakers with her at all times, you might be better off with both a handbag *and* a tote bag.

The Shoulder Bag

The alternative to the tote bag. This is a great bag to use when you're shopping, especially if you are multitasking and need to have your hands free. It's an absolute must-have. However, beware the little over-the-shoulder purse that some girls wear for dressy occasions—it crowds you, it detracts from the neckline of your garment, and it's basically for old ladies who don't want to be robbed.

The Duffel-Bag-Turned-Handbag

This is the bottomless-pit bag, the bag you fill with everything but the kitchen sink: shoes, a change of clothes, a water bottle, a toothbrush, toothpaste, you name it. Sizewise, this accessory is in between a weekend bag and a pocketbook, but it ends up looking and feeling like a duffel bag if it doesn't have easy-access compartments on the outside to hold your necessities, like your cell phone, wallet, keys, and sunglasses. This bag is ideal for a girl who walks out the door at nine in the morning and doesn't return until nine at night. I'm not opposed to a bag of this size, so long as you don't overutilize it and you choose a style that is slouchy and sloppy. It's kind of fun when it's slouchy and sloppy.

The Alligator Bag

Every girl should have one . . . or one that *looks* like real alligator. Alligator print is timeless and stunning, rich and slick, and it goes with *anything*, regardless of whether it's on a doctor's bag, a messenger bag, briefcase-style, or something softer.

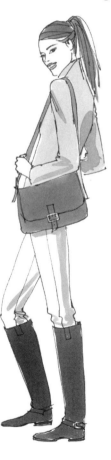

The Saddle Bag

This bag works great with chunkier jackets and blazers to create a fresh look. It's also a wonderful work bag *and* weekend bag. Perfect for the girl who is a pack rat, the saddle bag looks good whether it's bulky or flat. And the fact that it's designed to evenly distribute weight across the chest means less strain is put on the shoulders.

The Seasonal Bag

You can wear leather all year round, but you shouldn't wear suede in the summertime. A heavy, wintry fabric, suede is much less transitional, so you can't treat it like you would treat leather, and the same applies to embroidered bags and fur bags. On the other hand, straw and canvas bags are perfect for summer, and sequined bags can be worn all year long. In terms of color, go with brighter hues and pastels for the summer and saturated dual tones for the fall.

IT'S WHAT'S ON THE INSIDE THAT COUNTS: WHAT EVERY STAR-POWERED DIVA SHOULD CARRY IN HER PURSE . . . AND WHY

BLOTTING PAPER Even celebrities can't always have their makeup artists in tow. So when their skin is oily and they are between interviews or on the red carpet, they'll turn their heads, pull out the blotting paper, and dab themselves inconspicuously, like they're using tissue. The same trick will work if, say, you're out to dinner with a gentleman friend and you don't want to get up from the table to give yourself a quick touch-up. Just fake a sneeze and, with blotting paper in the palm of your hand, touch your face like you're ready to faint while secretly removing the shine in that cheek or brow area.

THE SEWING KIT THAT YOU TOOK FROM THE HOTEL Fashion emergencies happen. Okay, so Julia Roberts isn't likely to whip out her sewing kit and get busy in front of the flashbulbs and fans, but I've often put those cardboard-mounted kits in celebrities' bags before they hit the red carpet. That way, if something happens and I can't get to my celebrity client, she can go to the bathroom attendant and ask for help. In your case, if you have your trusty sewing kit, you can make the necessary adjustments yourself or enlist a friend to patch you up.

THE CELL PHONE Preferably covered in some kind of exotic skin or rhinestones.

"THE MULTIPLE" BY NARS This all-in-one makeup stick can be used on your eyes, cheeks, and lips, or as a body shimmer. It freshens up a face in seconds.

EXTRA TOPSTICK This double-sided tape is for the sexy girl who's wearing something a little bit daring. Especially essential if you're sweating on the dance floor.

A CREDIT CARD When cash is too bulky, this will do nicely. If you're a star, people should know who you are. And even if you're not, they should still know who you are. Flashing a credit card with your name on it is like saying, "Dial 411 and look me up."

✦ *If you don't have the luxury of buying a number of purses and bags in different colors, go for leather bags in neutral colors: black, brown, and camel, as well as metallics, mesh, and sequins. And while a red bag is not a necessity, don't shy away from bold colors. They can work like a neutral for a wardrobe that is filled with mostly the same colors. You'll actually be surprised at how well they mix with almost anything in your closet.*

The Judith Leiber Jewel-Encrusted Couture Purse

Almost like wearing a huge diamond solitaire, this is effortless glamour at your fingertips. Best when worn with a simple dress or gown, the Judith Leiber purse has definitely established its place in society. So if you can afford it, why not add it to your list of essentials?

The Evening Purse or the Clutch

Women often confuse clutches with purses. *Purses* are for more dressy occasions, whereas *clutches* have handles and are suitable for slightly more casual events. So, if you own either an evening purse *or* a clutch, you're good to go. And if you're not one to travel lightly, you can get a clutch that works for the evening, with enough room to store everything that the Girl Friday needs.

FOOTWEAR

It's common knowledge that every woman loves shoes. Shoes, after all, are *a girl's best friend*. You will collect far more shoes than diamonds during your lifetime, and you'll become far more attached to your footwear than your pocketbook. Shoes can take you from schleppy to sexy. They can right an outfit gone wrong, and they can change your posture as well as your attitude, instantly giving your legs a different silhouette. If you have big feet, a rounded toe can make them look smaller, whereas if you have small feet, a pointy-toed shoe will give you a little more length.

A woman often looks at a man's watch to get a sense of what kind of person he is. Well, these days a guy will just as often look at the kind of shoes a girl is wearing in order to get a read on her. Your shoes are your foundation, they keep you grounded, and they are the root of your look, the thing that can turn it around and give it a different vibe. That's why some women collect footwear. It's their hobby, and they have more shoes than they have outfits. In fact, you can give one outfit three different looks just by changing the shoes (or boots). Footwear is very accessible, and there are many options. However, there *are* a few essentials, a few pairs that you'll need no matter what, and that you can never spend too much money on.

✦ FOOTWEAR ESSENTIALS

Classic Closed-Heel Pumps
Pumps can be the foundation accessory for a casual outfit. Blue jeans were invented to be unfussy and easy, but think what you can do to glam them up—picture your favorite denims with a pair of diamond-studded pumps and a lace top. Now *that* is style.

Crystal Evening Shoes
These are your must-haves for evening glamour because they play well with both a gown and simple pants. Plain evening shoes, open-toed, open-heeled . . . take your pick—these will prove to be a great standby when you want to glam up any outfit.

✦ *If you have wide feet and want to wear strappy open-toed shoes, here's a celebrity style tip: Have your friendly shoemaker attach similar-colored elastic extensions onto the strap that connects to the sole.*

Wedges
A girl may not feel as sexy in a pair of wedges as she does in her stilettos, but there's definite compensation in the height and support that wedges

offer. They have become more and more stylized over the years, and there are even wedges designed for different seasons, whereas you used to see them only in the summertime.

Ballet Slippers or Driving Loafers

These are great if you're the type of girl who lives in pumps and can't wear sneakers unless you're going to the gym. It's a mental thing. Celebrities can be the same way. Even when they're feeling really schleppy, they'll put flip-flops on with cargo pants, a T-shirt, and a fur coat. They live in an exaggerated world where part of the fun is the ability to dress obnoxiously. The girl who loves driving loafers can also have extremely preppy taste. She might wear her loafers with slacks and jeans, is likely to have a wide variety of cashmere sweaters and pashmina scarves, and chances are she'll also own a great selection of watches and classic pocketbooks. If you're either girl, please try to do things in moderation.

Knee Boots and Shin Boots

Flat or with heels, knee boots always look great, regardless of your shape and pretty much regardless of your age. Just remember, the boots must be fitted to the calf. There's nothing worse than seeing a chicken leg in a baggy knee boot. If your boot is sagging, have it taken in by your shoe tailor. And if you have big calves, look for boots with stretch so they don't cut off your circulation. You can always insert elastic bands to give you more room, or ask your virtuoso shoe tailor to add eyelets, leather laces, and elastic gussets at the back to make them lace up. If you have really short legs, don't go for a boot that comes to the knee. Get a shin boot that will leave you more leg to work with.

✦ *A celeb's biggest fear is falling onstage—or on the runway, if she's a model. Their shoes always have marked soles or a permanent grip stuck to the bottom. You can ask your local shoe repair shop to fit grips to your soles. Or, if you are running late, take scissors or a knife to create a tic-tac-toe on a slippery new pair of shoes.*

Flip-Flops

These are so easy to pull off . . . as long as you're not wearing them to work, where they're really not appropriate. Otherwise, they're great leisure wear—great for getting pedicures, and you can mix and match them with some of your high-end pieces to tone them down.

MIXING AND MATCHING

If you're carrying a real designer bag, it's unlikely that you'll be wearing faux shoes. However, if you do want to wear a cheap pair of shoes, your investment should be in your outfit. An inexpensive outfit with an inexpensive pair of shoes is sure to get you busted.

One of the things that turns celebrities into major stars is their willingness to think outside the box. They're not afraid to wear a superstylish bag with a luxurious jogging suit or a fashion sneaker with a pair of casual slacks. Accessories bring luxury into your life. And when you don't have the disposable income to go all the way, style is all about the best compromise.

Always aware of the one thing that can become a conversation piece, celebrities and stylists often build outfits around a pair of shoes or a bag. Some celebs buy custom-designed shoes for publicity tours and big Hollywood nights, and entire outfits can be abandoned if they don't find the shoes and bags to match. That, my dear, is known as a *fashion crisis*! Still, don't feel pressured to keep up with celebrity shopping habits, because let me tell you, when stars fall in love with a bag or shoe, they'll wear it numerous times and feel no guilt.

On the following page are some ideas for mixing and matching shoes, bags, and outfits that will enable you to achieve true star power.

Wear pumps or, if you want a little more edge, go with platforms. By this
I don't mean seventies platforms. They would be too heavy and take away
from the classic quality, whereas a shorter platform will add a bit more
fun. For instance, a boot looks terrific with a classic dress and makes
it very edgy—picture Audrey Hepburn in a simple, high-neckline
cat-black dress with a pair of knee-highs and a low-waisted belt, or wearing a superfitted boot underneath a really full skirt. Platforms vary
in popularity from season to season, but they never go out of style.
They're perfect for the lady who loves the height and also needs a little
more sturdiness. Then again, an ankle pump looks great with an A-line
or fishtail skirt that has a little bit of swing. Add a bag and the look is
complete. If it's evening, you can take your clutch; if it's daytime, you can
wear your handbag.

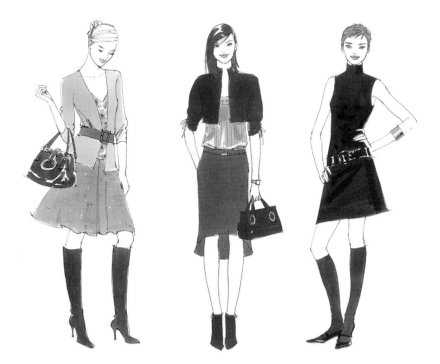

✦ If Wedges Are Your Thing

These are extremely sexy when you see lots of leg. They are the perfect solution for girls who've abandoned their pumps for something more comfortable. If embellished, wedges can look very ethnic, but whatever the look, they're invariably casual and campy. However, wedges are not an evening shoe of choice. Some supertrendy girls who are overstylized might wear wedges in the evening, but they're the exception to the rule. And since wedges are so campy, they go well with the sportier type of bag; something croissant-shaped, or a shoulder drawstring bag.

✦ If You Want to Add Some Energy to a Serious Suit

Wear a peep-toe shoe. Peep-toes are great because they're very transitional. You can wear them in the fall with some tights, and they'll move effortlessly into the spring and summer with bare legs. They make a corporate suit a little more fun without making you look inappropriately dressed—you're not displaying all of your toes, just a sassy bit of foot.

✦ *There's nothing worse than ill-fitting shoes that look borrowed, with either toe cleavage at the front or your hoofs hanging off the back.*

These are the first signs that you're in denial about the store not stocking your size. And you're also kidding yourself if you think opaque stockings or tights with open-toe sandals can be excused by claiming, "I forgot to get a pedicure," or "My toes are cold." Yeah, right. While open-toe shoes are great evening wear all year round, it's a totally different story if a celeb or anyone else puts them on in twenty-degree weather during the day. *Yuck!* Of course, you can bet your life it's been done, because some stars like nothing more than creating trends to confuse the fashion consumer—just think of the snow-boot-and-sundress look.

✦ If You Want to Strut Your Stuff in Classic Closed-Heel Pumps

These look terrific with a tight, fitted skirt suit because they're great day shoes, and when you wear them at night they'll go fine with jeans and a satin top. In both cases, take your pocketbook. This will transition perfectly from day into night as you replace your work blouse with your camisole. In this case, an earring change may come in handy as well.

✦ If It's Time for the Crystal Evening Shoes

These can be worn two ways: You can play them down with denim, or play them up with an evening dress. They're a great investment, and they add sparkle to the girl who's a minimalist and who doesn't have a lot of jewelry. The crystal evening shoes *are* her jewelry. Accordingly, pair them with a simple bag; not a crystal pocketbook, but a satin purse or a really clean-finished skin that will contrast with the crystals. Even if you're wearing an evening dress, go for a textured pocketbook over a diamond bag. You can get away with a diamond purse if you're attending a superglamorous event, but it would have to be something like a cruise ship dinner where you want to impress the captain.

✦ If That Flashy Judith Leiber Purse Deserves an Outing

It looks *beautiful* with a satin evening shoe, whether it's pointy, closed-toe, or open, but beware of putting it with jeweled footwear. You're featuring the purse, so don't upstage it. Your shoes should be very classic, very clean and simple, but they should still have great texture and be in a neutral color. Likewise, your outfit should be clean and elegant, without loads of ruffles or a busy pattern. The Judith Leiber is a beautiful evening bag as long as you don't wear things that try to compete with it. It's the star of the show and, as such, a surefire conversation piece.

✦ If You're Wearing a Kitten Heel or Casual Shoe

Go for a tote bag or something over the shoulder. This will create a cool, casual look for when you are in your mover-and-shaker mode. Kitten heels and nice, casual shoes will go great with trousers, slacks, summer skirts, T-shirts, and jeans.

✦ If It's a Day for Flip-Flops

Then it's also a day for the casual cotton or seersucker skirt that comes to the knee or down to the ankles, along with a summer tote, or a canvas or straw bag. Don't wear flip-flops with a miniskirt unless you're on the beach.

✦ *In the summertime, when you're wearing a brand-new thong or sandal, your feet tend to sweat. If they start to blister, spray them with deodorant. You get blisters because the skin breaks when it's moist, but you can avoid this if you keep your feet dry by spraying them with a powder deodorant.*

TIME TO REPAIR VERSUS TIME TO REPLACE

You can never predict what your footwear will have to endure once you leave the house. Before you wear a shoe, whether it's a Jimmy Choo or a Steve Madden, you should always have the soles reinforced to give your footwear a longer lifespan and save you the trouble of running to the shoe tailor after only the second wearing. You have to treat your shoes like they're puppies and really take care of them, because they are going for walks every day. Don't wear leather shoes in the rain—instead, change into your rain shoes. Your patent leather pumps could probably survive a shower, but their leather soles should still be treated before you expose them to bad weather. Scotchgarding will save you plenty of tears on a rainy day or after a messy meal that has spoiled your pair of pumps.

When the metal part of a heel is causing a *click-click-click* and it's skidding on the road, it is time to get your tire repaired. And when the toe of your shoe is looking kicked out and slightly eaten away, have it treated before the leather is completely destroyed. Leather shoes should be conditioned during the summertime along with anything else you plan to store, such as your boots. That way, they won't crack as fast. Nevertheless, when footwear has already been reinforced a couple of times and the base is split in two, get rid of it.

Many of the same rules apply to bags. When they start to crack and can't be conditioned or repaired, they should be tossed. A beaten-up old bag may work for men—such as a really worn doctor's bag that suggests experience—but a polished woman will never carry something that's cracked and worn out. Some bags are timeless and you don't ever want to get rid of them, and others are disposable and you just have to rotate them to ensure their longevity. Divas with star power know when to move on.

CHAPTER SEVEN

HAIR AND MAKEUP

A WOMAN

is never fully dressed until her nails have been polished and her hair and makeup have been done. That's why it's essential for you to complete the finishing touches. You don't have to go full-on RuPaul to brighten things up, but you do have to avoid bad makeup and lousy hair that can turn your chic look to shabby. That's like serving wonderful food with a rotten garnish—the presentation means everything.

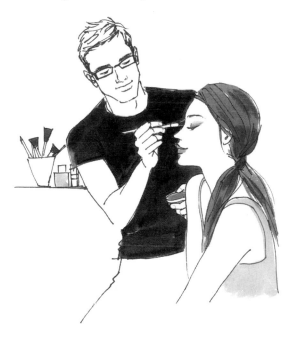

Your hair and makeup are just as important as your outfit, so you must have the full package in order to look your best. A great haircut and a well-made-up face have an enormous impact on your confidence level and your ability to feel and embrace all of the beauty that you already have. Hair and face maintenance is a huge part of taking care of yourself, so let's take a look at what you can do to complete your transformation without—or in addition to—resorting to cosmetic surgery.

HAIR

Unless you're determined to stick with a particular style, your hairstyle should be defined by the rest of your look. For example, if you dress sleek and slinky with plenty of black leather in your wardrobe, you don't want to start feathering your hair. You want something striking, like a ponytail, or a cut with great angles, like bangs and a bob. Then again, if your clothes are really soft and feminine, go for hair that has more layers, waves, and curls. Or, if you are into more of a retro look, your hair will look great if it's wavy, whimsical, and romantic.

Bangs and a blunt cut lend themselves to a very slick appearance and are a good look for a woman with edge; hair that is cut in layers and is very wispy suits a carefree woman who'll take those extra three minutes to style her hair. The type of woman who prefers slicked-back hair pulled into a ponytail is going to be very mod; and the woman who cuts her hair really, really short will indulge herself with plenty of fun colors and prints and a rambunctious silhouette, perhaps featuring big collars and lots of ruffles because her neck is exposed.

There are countless ways to get a look wrong by failing to style your hair to match your outfit, but the biggest faux pas is if your hair does not complement the shape of your face. So before you go to the salon, you may want to consider the following.

✦ If Your Face Is Long and Thin

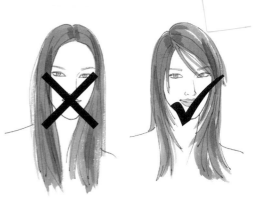

Stay away from straight-line styles that are all one length, because they will elongate your face. Instead, you should veer more toward a feathered cut with layers around the face that help to frame it, break up the lines, and give it more shape.

✦ If Your Face Is Heart Shaped

Go for styles that are full around the jawline and even out the face, making you look a little narrower in the forehead area and wider around the jaw.

✦ If Your Face Is Pear Shaped

Stay away from styles that frame the bottom of your face. You want more fullness on top, which means layering there while going for shorter hair around the sides and back of the head.

✦ If Your Face Is Round

Stay away from round styles such as bobs. You want to go for cuts that are all one length and fall below your shoulders; layered bangs are also great for this face shape.

✦ If Your Face Is Oval

You can get away with virtually anything, so let your personality dictate your hairstyle.

The position of your part also depends on the shape of your face, as well as which you consider to be your better side. (We *all* have a better side.) For instance, if you favor the left side of your face, then the part should be there, and vice versa. That's because it opens up the face and people's eyes will automatically go to that side.

HAIR MAINTENANCE

The way you wash and dry your hair plays a vital role in its overall look, and to that end you should bear the following in mind:

✦ If You Have Relaxed, Straight Hair

It tends to be dry and is more prone to tangling and breakage. Since it craves moisture, use supermoisturizing conditioner to keep it healthy, rinse your hair really well to avoid weighing it down, always use heat to dry it, and take your time combing when it's wet, as that is when the hair is most fragile. Use a powerful dryer with a nozzle to avoid burning the scalp, and hold it about a half inch from the hair. Dry in quarter-inch sections, and if you want a superstraightened look, use a really big, round brush or a comb that attaches to the dryer. Do this until the hair is three-quarters dry, and then continue to blow dry while randomly adding a shot of cold air every ten seconds or so to get more shine. The beauty of straight hair is that you can get incredible shine, and if you want to maximize your gloss, use a ceramic iron when straightening.

✦ If You Have Wavy Hair

Wavy hair tends to be a little dry as well, so use a leave-in conditioner that will coat the hair and enable it to dry with less frizz, and then let it dry naturally instead of using a blow-dryer. If you're in a hurry, use a diffuser, which will dry the hair quicker without making it frizzy. And if you still get some frizz on the surface, wrap unruly locks around a small curling iron to provide a better finish and give the impression that you've curled your entire head of hair.

✦ If You Have Curly Hair

Curly hair is generally even frizzier than wavy hair, so use a little more leave-in conditioner, as curly hair craves moisture too. Once again, let it dry naturally and curl flyaways.

These rules apply regardless of your hair color, although if you color your hair you must always use moisture-infusing shampoos and conditioners. L'Oréal has a wonderful line called Nature's Therapy, with Mega Moisture shampoo and conditioner that really soften, smooth, and revitalize processed hair.

HAIR FIXES

✦ IF YOU ARE TRYING TO GROW YOUR BANGS
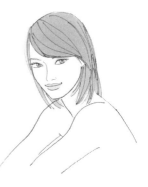
Pull hair from the sides of your face and sweep it over the bangs to make them look longer. I'm not asking you to sport a comb-over, but a deeper side part will help you cover up the short hair at the front. Or, if you prefer, wear your hair back and clip your bangs at the crown rather than emphasize the bangs by pulling them down.

✦ IF YOU NEED A COLOR TOUCH-UP BUT CAN'T GET TO THE SALON
Apply a color stick to your part and whatever other roots you can see. However, for best results, never recolor your own hair. Always see a professional.

✦ IF YOUR STRAIGHTENED HAIR CURLS DUE TO RAIN OR PERSPIRATION
Make sure you apply enough products before you leave the house. Products are your barrier against the natural elements, so use plenty of serum, conditioner, and/or gel, and distribute it evenly by combing it through your hair rather than just putting it on the surface. That way, you'll protect every strand.

✦ IF YOUR HAIR IS SUPERTHIN
Wigs and clip-on hairpieces are a must-have. A clip-on piece is also the answer to every bad hair day—wherever you are, you can pop it on and look better in an instant.

CHOOSING A HAIRSTYLIST

If you haven't already found a great stylist, one of the best ways of doing so is to ask someone whose cut really impresses you where she gets her hair done. A girl's do is her stylist's calling card. And you should always try to use people who specialize in certain areas; there are some who just cut hair, those who just style, and others who just color. Do your research, talk to people, and find the best hairstylists for every hair need. This is what most celebrities do. Just remember to follow the golden rule: Always have a picture as a reference. After all, your idea of short may not be the stylist's idea of short, and pictures are a great way of communicating.

✦ HAIR ALERT: *When you experiment with different styles, make sure you really love a particular look before you go all the way. You can always ask a stylist to take more off the length, but if the cut is too short, you can't perform an emergency reattachment. So tell your stylist to go slow. And before you cut or dye your hair, ask yourself, "Is this something I can live with?" If the answer is, "I don't know," ditch the scissors and toy around with wigs or clip-on extensions to add length, dimension, or volume. That way, you can make a drastic change, have hairstyles on the go, and nothing is permanent. Sure, really good wigs are expensive and extreme, but many big celebs are opting to use them instead of putting their natural hair through too much processing and hair drying.*

MAKEUP

Most big stars have makeup artists on call twenty-four hours a day and will even fly them in when there's a fashion emergency. These artists make tons of money and are well worth the cost—they save celebrities a fortune in plastic surgery. Rosacea, freckles, birthmarks . . . all of these complexion issues can be solved with makeup. Indeed, makeup should be like a second skin, but it should never be overdone, for while it can

help you to achieve a lot, the opposite is also true—using the wr
eye shadow and lipstick is a surefire way to destroy an outfit. V
eye shadow that matches your garment is an absolute no-no, becau
look contrived and campy, and the same goes for brow-bone highligh..crs
and severe, black, Marilyn Manson–style lip liner. You can also end up
making yourself look older or tired by selecting the wrong colors and
making mistakes during application.

Of course, some girls aren't into makeup, and some need less of it
than others—a woman with incredible skin might opt to use only
blushes and maybe some mascara. However, the fact is that most
women aren't makeup savvy at all. And because they don't know how
to choose or apply it, some won't go anywhere near it.

Ladies, don't be afraid of makeup. Every major department store has
makeup counters with experienced makeup artists who are there to help,
so talk with them and have them create a formula that caters to your
wants and needs. If, say, you want to wake up and look fresh and pretty
for the office, even though you have children and therefore can't spend
more than five minutes on your face, there's a formula for that. Indeed,
there are loads of great makeup regimens for people who are on the go as
well as for those who have all the time in the world. And while you can
spend $150 to $200 at a department store to get your makeup done for a
special event—a small price to pay for a finishing touch, especially if
you've already spent hundreds more on your shoes, dress, and bag—you
can also find plenty of makeup artists at the department store who will
do it for free if you purchase a few of the products and brushes.

If you're not makeup savvy, experimentation can lead to disaster.
However, don't be intimidated. Read the following tips, and for more
specific advice, visit your nearest department store.

AT WORK

Start with tinted moisturizer instead of foundation. Nowadays tinted
moisturizers contain many skin-saving ingredients, so they protect your

...n while giving you a nice glow. For example, there are lovely moisturizers from MAC on the market that provide sun protection, cover up blemishes, and even out skin just as well as any foundation.

Next, choose convertible colors—colors that will look good on your eyes, lips, and cheeks in natural light. A lot of makeup companies are now selling convertible colors either as part of a palette or in a tube. You can use them for eyes, lips, and cheeks, so with just two products your face is done. In addition, mascara and lip gloss are now often incorporated within space-saving makeup packages that are influencing women to become their own makeup artists, play with colors, and mix textures rather than just color by numbers.

IN THE EVENING
You can glam up your day look by perhaps going for a darker eye shadow on the lid, or using a lash liner as opposed to an eyeliner to intensify your lash line. Simply smudge it with your finger or a mascara wand to create a sultry look. Make sure to use short-handled brushes at home so that you're closer to the mirror. (Long-handled brushes are for artists to distance themselves a little from their subject.) Curl your lashes with the Shu Uemura industry-standard curler, the best one on the market, and apply mascara exclusively to the root, not from root to tip. This will make your lash line pop, and once the lashes have been curled they will look feathery if you don't apply mascara all the way to the tip. Then, for your lips, apply a natural gloss; feminine demarcation lines around the lips are to be avoided, so skip the lip liner. You can't go wrong with a more sophisticated, lacquered look.

FOR THE CLUB
Colorful eye shadows are very popular, as opposed to shimmering glitter that will date your look. Save the luminosity makeup for your body—shoulders, collarbones—and stick to sunny hues such as brown, bronze, and marigold. Dual tones, consisting of one base color and some iridescence

on top, are also big right now. And girls are really into fake eyelashes, which, when done right, can look supersophisticated. The trick with these is to use two sizes, because just one size will look unnatural. As for the lips, something with a rust undertone, like Spanish red or brick red, looks very sexy and will work regardless of your clothing or skin tone when you go for heavy definition around the eyes.

INDOOR VERSUS OUTDOOR

This is mostly about finish, whether it's matte (little to no shine), dewy (a moisture-rich shine), or satin (in between matte and dewy). Some girls prefer their makeup to look satiny, which works both indoors and outdoors. If, on the other hand, your finish is dewy, it's a great indoor look, but you'll run the risk of looking shiny when you go outside into natural light. As for matte-finish makeup, ensure that you incorporate some luminosity, using makeup with a little shimmer—if you only use matte makeup on your chin and under your eyes, you can be luminous on your temples, your cheeks, and your profile.

BEFORE APPEARING IN FRONT OF A CAMERA

Select an artistry line of makeup as opposed to a designer line. Artistry lines have been created either for professionals or for consumers by experienced makeup artists, and the results are formulas that are perfect in front of the lens. These artists definitely know what works well on camera, so go for lines like MAC, Stila, NARS, or Shu Uemura. They will provide you with a better payoff in terms of color because they're so highly pigmented, and you'll see better textures in the photographs.

The top designer lines aren't as rich as the artistry lines, and they're also more expensive, thanks to their prestigious names. Some of those manufacturers have recently been hiring fashion designers to formulate their lines, but although the colors are brilliant and beautiful, the results still aren't as good. What's more, if you purchase an artistry line at a cosmetics counter, nine times out of ten you'll receive better service because your retail artist is aspiring to become a celebrity makeup artist.

As they become incredibly popular, commercial lines like L'Oréal are now competing with artistry lines and introducing the likes of HiP (High-Intensity Pigments)—with its lip glosses, lip liners, lipsticks, and eye shadows—and True Match foundation, while Revlon has its own Color Stay foundation. These are as good as, if not better than, many of the artistry line products, and the same goes for mascaras that are readily available at most drugstores, such as Maybelline's Sky High Curves and its legendary Great Lash, as well as Volume Shocking and Voluminous by L'Oréal.

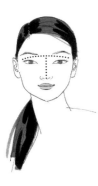

Of course, when you prepare for the camera, it's all about what will work with the lighting. And while it's difficult to be specific in this regard, a general tip is to always go for a matte finish on the T-zone. If you're contouring for photography, do so with cream concealers or cream foundations as opposed to powder ones. Powder eye shadows, in particular, create heavy demarcation lines and, in conjunction with your face's natural oils or the moisture of your foundation, enable the camera to pick up green, blue, red, and orange undertones.

FOR A HEALTHY GLOW

Add luminosity under your eyes and the C-Zones that run from your temples to your cheeks. Some beautiful, subtle contouring on the cheeks will add to the fresh-faced effect. If done properly, your face will look totally natural. All of which brings us to the most important makeup trick a girl should know: contouring.

Selecting the correct brush is vitally important, since this tool will do the work for you. You can pick up beginner brushes at any convenience store or drugstore, and once you get the feel for them, you can purchase more expensive brushes at higher-end stores. High-quality brushes will last ten years or more, so while they may be pricey, they're a worthwhile investment. For contouring, you might want to use a Kolinsky brush, whose bristles are soft, smooth, firm, and perfectly suited for shading. However, no matter what brand you select, be sure to go for bristles that are natural hair—goat, squirrel, or mink sable. These are less abrasive and create almost zero demarcation lines. Once you've used your brushes, wash them with your own shampoo and conditioner, and dry them flat as opposed to upright so that the water doesn't travel down to the part of the brush where the metal meets the wood and unravel the glue.

You want your contouring to appear completely seamless, and the best way to achieve this is to blend two or three colors in the same family, varying according to complexion. Here's how to approach the face.

THE CHEEKBONE AREA

Start with a concentration of color in the center of the apple of your cheek, and then blend outward and inward, going toward the temple—even lightly around the forehead—and back toward the bridge of your nose.

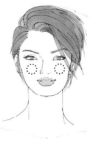

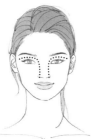

THE NOSE

The trick here is to start contouring from the outer corner to the inner corner of one eye, down the bridge of the nose, around the nostrils, and then from the top of the bridge to the inner and outer corners of the other eye. A lot of people contour the nose by making two straight lines down the center on either side of the bridge, but this just looks contrived, whereas if you blend seamlessly into the curve of the eyes, the end result looks completely natural.

UNDER THE CHIN

Create a shadow with shades that are slightly darker than your natural skin tone. Avoid heavy demarcation lines or a focus point by blending along the jawline.

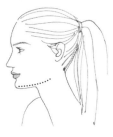

NAIL POLISH

On fingernails, it's always safe to go for neutral colors such as browns, beiges, or pinks that mimic your own flesh tone. However, you can still wear something brighter like a red or coral for a glamorous event, and the same applies to the toes. Your personality dictates your polish color choices. Feel free to experiment on your toes—make them as fun and loud as you like. Polish should be applied within the lines of your nails with smooth, even strokes. Never leave home with chipped nails—you'd look better with no polish whatsoever—and always keep a file in your purse.

MAKEUP FIXES

✦ To Bring Down Eye Swelling After a Long Night
People used to apply Preparation H under the eyes, and while this is a fine remedy, today there are plenty of products on the market specifically for-mulated to relax muscles and remove demarcation lines and wrinkles around the eyes. These include the same miracle ingredient as Preparation H—caffeine—but they don't bear the unpleasant smell. I recommend Freeze 24-7. Used topically, this product reduces fine lines, wrinkles, and swelling.

✦ If You Want to Whiten Reddish Eyes
Mavala Eye-Lites are amazing. These blue eye drops relieve the redness, and the yellowness as well, and they take effect immediately upon application.

✦ If You Have Wrinkled Eyelids

Apply a matte, sandy eye shadow to the skin and then use a shimmery shadow on top with an antique gold or silver finish. Never put shimmery makeup directly on mature skin, because that will only exacerbate the wrinkles.

✦ If You End Up with Eye Shadow Under Your Eye

Don't try to remove the misplaced makeup. Instead, clean it up with foundation or tinted moisturizer, ensuring that you correct the mistake without disturbing what's underneath.

✦ If You Have Thin Eyebrows

Start in the center of the eyebrow, right above the pupil, and with an eyebrow pencil create angular lines across the top of the eyebrow and then round lines toward the bottom, blending the color outward before focusing on the fine line at the outer corner. Never start at the inner point of the eyebrow (nearest the eye) to create a demarcation line. The effect is too severe.

✦ If You Apply a Lipstick with Heavy Pigmentation and Then Want to Change the Color

Because there's such a heavy color deposit in the original shade, it'll mix with whatever you put on top. However, to completely erase the bottom color, apply foundation and powder to the lips and then redo the color. Your lipstick should be chosen based on what you're wearing and your natural lip color. When a girl finds a texture and a color she really likes, she'll often stick with it like it's her favorite fragrance and become a creature of habit with that one product. Nevertheless, lip wear should always change with your mood and your outfit.

✦ If Your Makeup Looks Too Dewy

Use a synthetic film that will absorb all of the oil without disturbing your makeup. Johnson & Johnson's Clean & Clear is the best product on the market.

There are plenty of lip plumpers on the market right now, and Freeze 24-7's PlumpLips is probably the best. What this product does is create a small allergic reaction that constricts the blood flow to your lips, and while it may sound weird, it isn't detrimental to your health. You'll have a sexy pout within a matter of minutes, and it'll stay that way for several hours. Then, if need be, you can reapply the plumper when your lips start to deflate.

TOOLS AND ACCESSORIES

These days, proper makeup bags look pretty much like cocktail bags or evening clutches. They have room not only for your makeup, but also for your touch-up kit, your brushes, your credit cards, and, in some cases, even your cell phone, and they are available everywhere.

The right tools are essential to makeup application. The best device you can use for applying foundation is your finger. There's not a brush on the market that's as warm as your finger, which heats up the makeup and enables it to spread nicely. That's why you can pretty much do your entire face with a mascara wand, lipstick, and your fingers. However, if you prefer to employ a sponge and you need more coverage, be careful with latex. A lot of girls are allergic to it, but they often attribute their reaction to the makeup rather than the instrument that they're using.

Also, a lot of foundations now have silicone, which might interfere with latex sponges, so stay away from sponges if at all possible; use your finger, and buff with a synthetic foundation brush. Buffing is very important to ensure that your lines are seamless, there are no demarcation lines, and you have a porcelain-smooth application.

There is so much room for error when it comes to putting on your face. While some mishaps are painfully obvious—clown makeup, clumpy eyelashes—there are also some that are less noticeable, at least to the perpetrator. . . .

✦ APPLYING CONCEALER BEFORE THE FOUNDATION

If you apply heavy concealer before foundation, the foundation is not likely to stick to the concealer. Applying more concealer is futile, as it won't stick either. As a result, when you apply powder, there's such a heavy concentration of concealer already caked on the skin that the powder will shift on the concealer and appear discolored compared to the rest of your face. Apply tinted moisturizer or foundation first, and *then* reach for the concealer.

This applies to under-eye concealer as well—it should always be applied *after* foundation or tinted moisturizer. The silicone-based concealers are incredible compared to cream- or water-based formulas; silicone never permeates the skin but floats on top of it, filling fine lines and wrinkles and making them disappear.

✦ OVERWORKED EYEBROWS

These end up looking like threads, with no shape whatsoever. Eyebrows are important to a woman's face—they can open it up, lengthen it, widen it—so never work on your own eyebrows unless you've mastered using a pencil, brow groomer mascaras, and tweezers.

If you don't feel comfortable working on your own eyebrows, go to a local beauty salon or an eyebrow threader and let the artist take his or her time with one eyebrow while you give direction. Start off slowly, taking care of one row at a time, and get the shape absolutely right before moving on to the next eyebrow. Afterward, when everything is to your satisfaction, take a photo of the results so that you always have a point of reference.

This does happen. Water-based products like mascara will go bad within two to three weeks and serve as a breeding ground for bacteria. So make sure you replace your mascara as often as possible and open it only for application. Also, if you have silicone-based products, don't store them in places that are too cold, just like you don't want to store cream products in places that are too hot.

AGE-BASED MAKEUP

The universal rule of makeup application is to highlight your best feature and downplay the rest. When done right, makeup can give you an incredible psychological boost. It can make you feel young and sexy, and it doesn't require going under the knife. Older women should focus on that part of the face with the best skin, matting it down and applying a silicone highlighter on top. Likewise, if you have really nice eyelids while the rest of your face is mature, focus on those, and do the same with your lips if they're plump and beautiful. Just concentrate on your most flattering feature and play it up.

Teenagers should definitely focus on toning, cleansing, and moisturizing their skin. And in this regard Johnson & Johnson's Clean & Clear line is a must—this has Blackhead Clearing Scrub, Blackhead Clearing Astringent, and Oil-Free Dual-Action Moisturizer. Also, L'Oréal has Ideal Balance Foaming Cleanser, Ideal Balance Pore Clarifying Toner, and Visibly Clean Foaming Cream Scrub Cleanser, while Cetaphil offers moisturizing cream and face wash. Then again, if you're a middle-aged woman who's in a transitional stage with your style, the best thing you can do is focus on your skin and cheekbones, making them radiant and dewy and supple. This will give you a fresh, sophisticated look.

✦ *Makeup can truly change the shape of a face and play tricks on the naked eye. Many celebs employ all kinds of tricks to look their best when they don't necessarily feel like glamour queens. Take, for example, the quickie eyelift attained by pulling the face back via thread glued to the temples and run through the hair to the back of the head. The thread is like fishing wire, and you can't see it because it's part of some flesh-colored lace material that is attached to the forehead and covered with makeup. This is one of the oldest tricks in the book—Lucille Ball used to employ it, and it's a regular practice in drag clubs—but oh, my dear, it works fabulously, like a mini facelift.*

BODY MAKEUP

Body makeup is a wonderful way to enhance your figure. This includes tanning solutions that are far less damaging to the skin than lying in the sun for hours and hours. Bronzing sticks are also must-haves, especially when you're wearing something with an open neckline—in addition to creating the illusion of sun-kissed skin, you can also craft muscles and definition or employ simple contouring in the chest area to make your breastbones protrude a little more. Body makeup is beautiful because it really adds nice texture and sheen to the skin, which is the first thing you take care of before you start to dress. It's your template.

Most women don't appear to realize that there are numerous face-and-body foundations on the market, and you can buy them in a variety of tones to contour and highlight the body. Stay away from products that contain high levels of oil, because it will transfer onto your clothes and it will move on the skin and appear blotchy. Airbrush foundations in aerosol cans are genius . . . so long as you remember to spray before you dress. And make sure you spray on your foundation in a bathroom where there's ceramic and porcelain, which can be easily wiped off.

If it's the dead of winter and you miss your summer glow, you can always visit your local tanning salon and get a spray-on tan. This can be very healthy for your skin if the tanner contains lots of vitamins and minerals. There are also multiple coloring sticks that can be really good for the body if you crush them and blend them into a moisturizer. Use this mixture to highlight your collarbone for more definition, and if you use a shimmering pigment such as a champagne or silver, this will intensify the color of your tan. Regular bronzing powder for the face is also gorgeous on the body *after* you've moisturized it.

Overall, when trying to decide on the makeup that works for you, it might be wise to visit a department store and consult various artists at the cosmetics counter. That way, you'll get different opinions and be able to create a palette of those looks—instead of buying single eye shadows, for example, you can purchase a palette with a gradation of browns, a palette with a gradation of purples, a palette with a gradation of reds, and on and on. Try different lines for different textures. And before buying an eye shadow for the color, make sure that you love the way it feels and the way it applies to your skin.

✦ *Always drink a lot of water to keep your skin moist and allow your makeup to last. Otherwise, when you are dehydrated, your skin will crave moisture and absorb your lip gloss, your blusher, your foundation, your eye shadow, and anything else you've applied. Remember, hydration and moisturizing are two different things. Hydration is water for your skin, while moisturizing is more like food for your skin.*

CHAPTER
EIGHT

FITS, FIXES, AND TRICKS OF THE TRADE

HAVE you ever noticed that celebrities always seem to fit perfectly into their clothes? Well, it's not because they all have perfect bodies. (Believe me; I've seen a lot of them naked.) The fact is, they actually have the same flaws as the rest of us. They're just better at hiding them.

There's nothing worse than people who don't recognize their flaws and torture themselves by strangling their bodies in smaller garments that don't necessarily fit, hoping to lose the excess weight in a week. Not only does this result in stress for the wearers, but they also end up with visible stress to their clothes in the form of back fat, rolls that don't exist, and the dreaded uni-breast.

If your weight has a tendency to fluctuate, you must be conscious of this and dress accordingly. A lot of my clients are aware that, at a certain time each month, they can increase by an entire dress size from one week to the next because of water retention. Therefore, they have clothes that allow for the expansion. And so should you. Buy garments that provide you with room to maneuver, not the motivation to diet.

You should also understand that your body is naturally asymmetrical. One breast is larger, one shoulder is higher, one leg is longer, and while this is subtle in many cases, some people don't recognize that the disparities are natural and simply assume that they're ill-shaped or

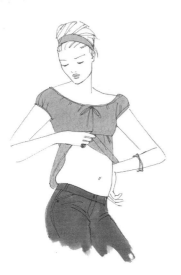

wearing the wrong size. That's why you have to really get to know your body, learn to love it for what it is, and dress accordingly.

With this in mind, pick the right time of month to shop. You don't want this to be when you're feeling fat or frazzled because your estrogen level is out of control. Even the easiest decisions might seem difficult, and the result could be an investment in clothes that you really don't need and, worse still, that really don't fit.

It's good to set goals for yourself so long as they're not unrealistic—buying a size six dress when you're a size ten will only result in the garment collecting dust at the back of your closet. Why not go for the size that you normally buy and then let your tailor take care of whatever you lose? It's usually going to be just a few inches rather than two or more dress sizes, unless you've bought a garment that you're planning on wearing in a year's time. Otherwise, not only will you have difficulty squeezing into that new acquisition, but if you do manage the feat you'll only emphasize the fact that you *are* oversize and draw attention to those extra bulges. So avoid a fashion disaster by camouflaging those areas that you either haven't finished tweaking or that are still under construction.

Dark, solid colors are ideal for creating silhouette and shape. Black absorbs light and hides imperfections while outlining the shape of the body. Other dark colors will also do. Just stay away from lighter tones and shinier fabrics that will bring attention to your problem areas. And don't shy away from alterations. A good tailor can work miracles.

HOW TO DISCERN A GOOD OR BAD FIT

Should you rely on the judgment of your friend-cum-fashion-consultant? Or should you take the salesperson's word for what looks good? These are both viable options—you can always tell that overenthusiastic salesperson or friend, "Look, if I get home and my husband doesn't like it, or if someone looks at me funny, I'm gonna bring it back." A simple threat may prompt the truth. The last thing he or she wants is a return.

However, it would still be best if *you* know what to look for and make your own decisions. With no one to blame but yourself, you're more likely to buy what's right. Just train your eye to look for certain imperfections, such as the following problem-causers.

✦ SIDE SPILLS
Anything that's pinching you in, cutting off your circulation, or causing extra ripples is just not worth it.

✦ A SAGGY OR OVERTIGHT CROTCH
Extra fabric that sags around the crotch is just not ladylike, whereas bunched-up fabric stretched across the crotch will overemphasize that you're a girl. It's also unattractive to see the seat of your pants sucked between the cheeks of your butt.

✦ BUTT-CRACK CLEAVAGE
This may be fashionable among some young girls, but there's nothing flattering about seeing someone's butt hanging out of their jeans. Also, denim starts to give after a while, the jeans get a little baggy, and the butt-crack cleavage becomes deeper as time goes along. That having been said, when trying on jeans you should ask the salesperson how much they will stretch, as well as how much they will shrink after the first wash.

✦ Squeezing of the Hips

If your skirt is bunching up in the crotch region, it does *not* fit. Ditto the stretchy off-the-shoulder dress that is pulling in all the wrong areas, including across the bust. This is not a good look.

✦ Gripping Underneath the Armpit

If you're trying on, say, a scoop-neck top, make sure it doesn't look like it's choking the armpit and causing a gather. That's a sure sign that the top does not fit you because your shoulders are too broad for it.

✦ The Top-Heavy Look

If a boxy, short-waisted jacket makes your shoulders look twice as wide, don't leave the store with it, even if it makes your waist look really small. You'll look like a linebacker.

✦ Bra Spillage

Look for back cleavage bursting out of a bra and your breasts pouring over the sides or out the top. These are the signs of a bad fit. Visit a lingerie store and have a saleswoman determine your correct size.

✦ Back Fat

Strapless gowns and dresses with spaghetti straps may pinch in the back and cause flesh to hang over the top. If you see this happening when you try on dresses, focus on low-cut fronts and high backs.

✦ Panty Lines

There's nothing worse than visible panty lines. They are a surefire way to destroy a chic look. Unless you're into fancy thongs, go for a covered bottom that doesn't hit you in the midcheeks. It should either be cut high on the waist, leaving very few lines and seams, or you should opt for French lace boy-style shorts where the lace is flat and doesn't leave an imprint. The indentation can also be caused by underwear that's too tight, or a thick band serving as finishing on the edges. At the same time, saggy bloomers aren't sexy either, because you can see them under fabrics or peeking out the tops of your pants and skirts. A seamless brief is perfect underneath an A-line skirt, while a low-rise brief plays well with a low-rise pair of jeans.

FIXES

✦ IF YOU HAVE SAGGING BREASTS

Do you ever wonder how your favorite star's breasts look perfectly perky and stay in place no matter what she wears, while yours tend to look lopsided and droopy? Sure, a lot of celebs get implants, but many also have some tricks up their sleeve (or down their blouse) that you can copy at home.

First and foremost, get yourself some great lingerie. Not the frilly, sexy stuff that you wear for your boyfriend, but sturdy, supportive stuff that will hide your flaws and add oomph where you need it as well as camouflage where you don't. As far as color goes, your best bet is nude. A lot of people think white bras should be worn under white T-shirts, but a white bra will actually show through the fabric, whereas nude lingerie is invisible.

Secondly, get yourself some chicken cutlets, and not the kind you find in Whole Foods Market. These are silicone implants that go inside your bra rather than under your skin, and they look a lot like the chicken breasts you cooked for dinner last night. They'll add lift to even the saggiest boobs. Why splurge several thousand bucks on implants when you can achieve the same effect with chicken cutlets for about twenty dollars?

Third, you can install bras into certain dresses. Just have the cups sewn onto the front of the dress rather than the entire bra. That way you'll avoid pinch at the back while inconspicuously gaining support at the front.

✦ IF YOU HAVE A SMALL CHEST

Either play it up or live with it. Select tops with a lot of gathering and ruching—the more detail, the better, although you can also make the most of your small chest by going for really low, plunging necklines, as daring and as deep as possible. Low-cut tops look really amazing on small-chested girls because they need no support, and wearing a tank top without a bra is tomboy sexy. Just make sure that if you wear a low, plunging top, it is fitted and lies flat. A roomy top on a flat-chested woman has the same effect as a six-year-old wearing her mother's clothes.

✦ If You Have Sagging Shoulders
Add shoulder pads by disassembling a jacket's inner lining and placing the pads on the underside of the fabric. Hand-stitch or pick-stitch the pad in place about an eighth of an inch off the shoulder so it protrudes just past the natural slope to give it some edge.

✦ If You Have Small Shoulders
Again, shoulder pads are an obvious solution, but sometimes it's better to remove them from outfits, because they're too wide and they look unnatural. In those cases I replace them with a thinner pad that better complements the wearer's shape. A jacket *can* have too much structure. Ruffle shirts and rope-shoulder jackets are two more stylish options that look great on girls who have narrow shoulders.

✦ If You Have Big Breasts and a Small Rib Cage
Taper through the upper part of the armhole. This will reduce excess fabric and leave you with a cleaner look. And again, if you want to dress a little sexier, remember that a bra can always be taken apart and sewn into a dress, tube top, or halter top to keep it in place, providing a clean, inconspicuous look and some much-needed support. Of course, if these options sound too technical, there's always good old gaffer tape—lift the breast and place one strip vertically underneath the boob to give it natural lift.

✦ If Nipples Are a Concern
Most women would rather show cleavage and the sides of their breasts than have their nipples piercing through a tight T-shirt. However, if you are among the nipple-phobic, don't worry about getting one of those fancy nipple petals. Just cover up with a good old Band-Aid. If, on the

other hand, you want to emphasize the impression of nipples protruding through a dress, you can buy specialized rubber imitations that stick to your skin. They're surprisingly lifelike.

✦ If You Have Wide Hips and a Small Waist
You'll need to go up two pant sizes and then recut the waist of the pants. It's almost like creating a piece from scratch—you're redoing the seat, taking in the waist, and bringing the crotch up; it's a major alteration, but one hundred percent worthwhile.

✦ If You Have a High Butt that Sticks Out
There are pants that'll not only work for you, but will look fabulous after a few alterations. Give them a long rise if they don't already have one and let out the seat. Then, if you're still self-conscious, wear long jackets to cover the problem area.

✦ If You Have a Thick Waist and Small Legs
Buy smaller pants to get a snug fit around the legs and then add a gusset or change the waistband altogether, substituting an elastic band that stretches but still holds the pants around the waist. No one has to know—just wear a blousy top that hides the waistband.

✦ If You Have a Beautiful Waist and Love Button-Down Shirts, but Hate the Blousy Shapelessness of the Cut
Place darts in the front and the back of the shirt, giving it a clean, sharp finish that allows you to showcase the stomach you've worked so hard to sculpt.

✦ If You Have a Broad Back and Wide Shoulders
Your biggest difficulty is finding jackets that fit. Your tailor can attack the problem by opening up the back seam and using the seam allowance to give you a little more room. And if you still need more room after that, add gussets using the same fabric, taken from an inconspicuous area of the jacket; perhaps under the lapel or an inside panel. This technique can

also be used for the side gussets. The result will be more room in the chest area and across the back. Meanwhile, another simple solution is to have the buttons moved—this will give you more room to breathe, and it's a nearly invisible alteration when done right.

DIY FIXES

These little beauty tricks will save you time and a trip to the tailor.

✦ If Your Ball Gown Has a Crinoline Netting Underneath that Has Lost Its Shape
After sitting in your closet for days on end, it probably won't have the grand appearance that you were hoping for. Don't panic. Just turn the dress upside down, shower it with holding hairspray, and then hit it with a hair dryer. *Et voilà,* your gown is now ready for the red carpet!

✦ If Your Garment Is Extremely Minimal or Unstructured
Use double-sided tape to keep it glued to your body so that you can actually walk in it. This is the best and most inconspicuous adhesive around—you won't see it even on the most delicate of fabrics. Every girl should use this miracle product to avoid having a boob pop out while she's gyrating on the dance floor.

✦ If You Want to Make a Pair of Jeans Your Own
Put them on, sit in a tub of warm water, and watch them contour to your body. Then just hang them and let them drip-dry naturally.

✦ If You Want to Prevent Static Cling on Your Tights or Stockings
Hairspray, Scotchgard, and dryer sheets are the obvious solutions, but if you really want some stylist trade-secret magic, put hand lotion on them. At least you're more likely to have this in your bag.

✦ If You Love Your New Pumps but Want to Cut Off Your Feet After Wearing Them for an Hour

Dr. Scholl's insoles and jelly pads are well-known remedies, but a lesser-known one is to put moleskin in the areas that are irritating you, such as the heel or the instep. This'll give you nice, padded, flesh-tone protection.

✦ If You Have Leather Shoes that Need Breaking In

This can be easily dealt with if you have the patience to wear them around the house with a pair of wet sweat socks for a few hours.

ALTERATIONS

A stylist will never put a client in something that's ill fitting. And although *you* may not have the will or the way to drop thousands of greenbacks on a couture gown or custom-made suit, you can certainly spend a few dollars on a skilled tailor. When you buy an outfit, regardless of its price tag, you can make it look far more expensive just by having it expertly altered so that it hangs like an Armani. This applies to every body shape.

Some people must have everything altered, whether they're oversize or petite. If you love a garment but it doesn't fit perfectly in the store, buy the item closest to your size and take it to the tailor. However, for best results, you don't want the alterations to be too drastic. If you must make changes, stick to tweaking the hem or the waist. It's particularly difficult to change the overall size of a pair of pants—sometimes you're better off just giving them away.

Letting out fragile fabrics like silk, rayon, velvet, and leather can also be a disaster—they are so delicate that, once a needle goes through them, the scars are permanent. Labor-intensive jobs like reshaping a lapel or taking in a neck can also be horror stories. So be realistic when you purchase things and then have them contoured to your body, especially when you're buying mass-market clothing but want everything to look like it's *prêt-à-porter*.

Of course, alterations aren't always about getting the perfect fit. I have taken pieces from past collections and remixed them so that you couldn't recognize the original garments. This is a great trick for when you have something that was purchased for a special occasion, such as an expensive prom dress or an elaborate bridesmaid frock, and that you'd like to make more practical for everyday wear. So if you think you'll get more use out of something by shortening it, removing the sleeves, or adding lace embellishments, a slip, or a bustier underneath, go for it!

PAYING FOR ALTERATIONS

Here are the kinds of per-job prices that you should expect to fork over in order to achieve a perfect fit.

Pant hems: $10 to $20

Skirt hems: $15 to $40

Sleeve hems: $8 to $25

Jacket alterations: anywhere from $40 to $150, depending on how labor-intensive the alterations are

Shoulder narrowing or resetting: $50 to $125

ALTERATION HAZARDS

You have to be selective in terms of the alterations that you choose to do, or else you and your unwitting garment will draw attention for all the wrong reasons. And you'd also be wise to leave well enough alone if a job is so costly or time-consuming that you might as well buy a new outfit. Turning a single-breasted jacket into a double-breasted jacket, taking ruffles out of a shirt if you're a big-chested girl—these kinds of jobs really aren't worth the effort.

Of course, it should be noted that certain clothes are easier to alter than others. For instance, raising an armhole is tough, as is lengthening a sleeve or a trouser leg when there isn't sufficient material to play with. The same goes for letting out a waist when there isn't enough give. Then there are the items that just aren't worth saving. A sure sign that a garment falls into this category is when it has torn in places other than the seams, or when your jeans have lost their elasticity. Jeans naturally stretch, but when they're stretching four or five different ways, it's a wrap. Some people like it when their jeans look worn and broken-in, but a broken-in look depends more on the wash than the fit. The same applies to sweaters that have lost their shape at the bottom and can't be taken in or rewoven. It's time to say adios.

LOOKING GOOD FOR A PHOTO SHOOT (OR FOR ANY DAY YOU NEED TO LOOK YOUR BEST)

This is all about advance preparation. Every day, as you get dressed, imagine that you're preparing to go in front of the camera or walk the runway. Then, when the time does approach for your own red carpet event or photo shoot, you'll be relaxed and ready, thanks to months of practice. However, if you're planning on wearing a tight dress, *please* don't have a plate of French fries or eat a bowl of pasta right before the event. Avoid foods that will bloat you, and drink plenty of water.

If possible, try on your entire outfit the day before to see if everything works and to determine whether you need to make any additions or changes. You don't want to wait until the cameras are about to flash or your partner says, "Honey, let's go," to realize that you don't have the right purse or the right earrings.

When selecting your wardrobe, don't choose *anything* that requires constant pulling, tugging, or fixing. This includes everything from your clothes and accessories to your hair and makeup. And if the photo shoot is taking place outdoors, have a Plan B in case of climatic changes or plain old bad weather. For instance, bring a patent leather skirt instead of a suede skirt, or a portable rain hat that can fit in your purse and save your hairdo at the last minute.

One of the things I always tell my celebrity clients the day before they pose in front of the lens is, "Go home and get some rest." Well, the same applies to you. In order to avoid feeling cranky and looking puffy, your body needs to recharge, and you can achieve that by drawing a mineral bath and applying moisturizers and essential oils. Honey, there's *nothing* like a massage and facial to make you feel like a star. And that star attitude, along with subtle makeup, the right clothes, and accessories, will help you feel flawless.

Of course, you're not going to be flawless—there's no such thing—but *feeling* flawless gives you the confidence that enables you to look in a three-sided mirror without fear. Now *that's* a beauty trick worth learning.

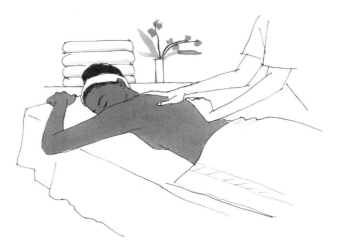

CHAPTER
NINE
ORGANIZING YOUR WARDROBE

LIKE your clothes, your closet reflects who you are. An organized closet belongs to an organized person, and if its contents are accessible to you, then life's opportunities will be endless and accessible too. So think of your closet as sacred ground. When you open it, you should feel like it holds the secrets to how your day is going to turn out.

The real world is a battle, and a clean, tidy, and well-organized closet will help make you the victor. There are numerous ways to achieve this goal. Find one that works for you and stick to it. The result will be that you feel happy and clear-minded about getting dressed in the morning, rather than frantic because you can't find your favorite cashmere sweater for the third time this month.

While all my celebrity clients have walk-in closets, even the most modest wardrobe can be organized to help you easily plan your look each day. First, get a good selection of clothes hangers by visiting www.hangers.com on the Internet or your local Container Store. You'll feel like your wardrobe is much more exclusive if all of your hangers match. And those free wire ones from the dry cleaners don't count! They are the worst thing you can do to your garments, because they'll misshape or even puncture your clothing. Likewise, if you have those plastic hangers with metal clips, don't attach your pants to them unless you have foam or tissue paper to protect the garment from snagging or being left with major lines. I've even seen some people fold their pants in two and clip them at the knees; not a good idea. They should either be draped over a hanger that has a little bit of grip to prevent them from slipping, or a pant hanger that has a rubber strap to hold them in place.

Hangers with little hooks are wonderful for tops and dresses that have very wide shoulders and can be attached by strings on the inside. Nevertheless, don't overlay garments on the same hanger—this might seem like a great space-saving idea, but it results in creased clothes that are hard to access and difficult to see. And the same goes for shirts and tops that are stacked on shelves. Keep everything as visible, accessible, and wrinkle-free as possible.

Having invested in some quality hangers, next divide up your clothes according to season—if it's summer, for instance, put all your sweaters and wool pants into storage, and repeat the process with your shorts and swimsuits when it's winter. Well, *most* of them, because there are pieces that you should hold on to in case of unforeseen weather conditions or travel to locales that have a different climate. That is why it's always worth keeping at least a couple of swimsuits at hand.

Layering pieces—such as T-shirts—are transitional; fur coats, cable-knit sweaters, and other heavy, chunky items are not. Neither are ultra-skimpy garments and any other very season-oriented clothes. These should be placed in storage to create closet space for current seasonal garments. Lightweight cashmere clothes don't have to be put in storage because they can be used all year round. They feel great in the spring and fall, can be used as layering pieces in the winter, and sometimes can even be worn on cooler summer evenings.

Storing items also depends on where you live. New York, for example, with its hot summers and freezing cold winters, experiences far greater variations in temperature than Los Angeles, where it's cold for only a few weeks each year and the residents therefore have little need

for many winter clothes. Those of you who live in place
clearly defined seasons should start packing away the no
pieces just before the major change in weather comes. Th
the temperature climbs or falls, you won't be caught unpr
next season arrives ahead of schedule.

Now, if you live in a one-bedroom apartment, have limited closet
space, and can't really afford outside storage, get creative finding close-
to-hand solutions to stow things away; under the bed in readily available
low storage containers, for example, or high in the linen closet, using
handy vacuum-sealed bags to remarkably compress your clothes—from
sweaters to goose-down coats—and take up the minimum amount of
room.

Still, smart storage is not just about convenience. If knits aren't stored
properly—neatly folded with tissue paper between the creases in cloth
boxes or in vacuum-packed bags—they'll look worn and may easily rip
when you pull them out next year. What's more, a good dry cleaner can
screen your white garments with a deoxidizing agent that will prevent
them from turning yellow when they're stored.

ORGANIZATION IS THE KEY

Once your closet contains only the seasonal garments you need, the next
step is to divide the tops and bottoms and then categorize them according to color (the *dominant* color when it comes to patterned and multicolored items). Color coding is really helpful, especially if you graduate
your tones; from whites to powder blues to grays to black and so on, like
day to night, sunrise to sunset. Space permitting, you can also divide fur-
ther based on work and play clothes. For example, keep one side of your
closet reserved for, say, skirts and suits that you wear to the office, and
the other side for your nights and weekend garments. This should be
possible for even a tiny closet, because unless you're a real nighttime
party animal or have a very relaxed work environment, the majority of

wardrobe will be dedicated to day wear, with a smaller section for leisure. The goal is never having to *hunt* for a particular item. An organized closet will reward you with invaluable time and readily available options.

STORING UNDERWEAR, LINGERIE, SHOES, AND ACCESSORIES

If possible, underwear and lingerie belong in drawers. However, many people can't afford closets with built-ins, and thus some are limited to just a shelf and some hanging space. If so, lingerie should be draped over sleeker hangers that aren't too bulky, while your underwear is placed in open-faced boxes on a specially designated area of the shelf, or in a simple dresser that, with drawer dividers, will help neatly display your panties, bras, and socks.

Ideally, shoes should be stored in a separate closet or cupboard with your pocketbooks and accessories, because otherwise you're putting the things that you use to walk on the streets next to things you're putting up against your skin. If you don't have the separate space, always store your shoes on the floor below your clothes, not above, in order to avoid having dirt fall down onto the garments. Either way, I recommend the use of shoe horns and boot braces to ensure that your footwear retains its shape. And like your clothing, shoes should be organized together for evening, business day, and athletic and casual.

Accessories should be separated in clearly visible drawer containers. Keep earrings with earrings, necklaces with necklaces, bracelets with bracelets, and so on for easy accessibility. And if you're really super-organized, put them in labeled containers. But whatever you do, don't throw all your jewelry into one box—that's the quickest way to tangle or ruin your collection. As for hats and scarves, they should be put into storage boxes and placed inside your *coat closet*—unless we're talking about a chic fashion hat that you can wear indoors.

CLOSET NO-NO'S

+ Placing furry items next to cashmere pants, or your cream mohair sweater next to your black trousers, causing major speckling and fuzziness. Linted garments are an easily prevented eyesore.

+ Hanging long dresses from a low shelf, scrunching up jackets, and hanging things on hooks that will create doggy ears or humps in the back.

+ Using those nasty mothballs that create such a stench and make you smell like you've visited a hospital. Scented sachet sacks are a whole lot nicer, and periodically airing your closet is also a good idea.

+ Leaving your dry-cleaned clothes in polyethylene bags for long periods of time. The clothes oxidize and acquire yellow stains that can never be removed. Fabric fiber needs to breathe.

+ Holding on to clothes that never get worn. Like a relationship that's not working, you need to ignore the separation anxiety and get rid of it. The valuable closet real estate will be better served by items you love. You won't regret it. Of course, if it's a perfectly good garment, give it to a consignment shop or donate it to charity, because there's always another body waiting for that piece. As the saying goes, your trash is somebody else's treasure.

THE SHELF LIFE OF CLOTHES

It's important to recognize when your good clothes have gone bad, and whether or not they can be saved. For instance, black has a limited shelf life because it's inevitable that it will turn to gray . . . unless it's a really rich black in a cotton cashmere fabric that has a strong luster. You can also keep a pair of black trousers for a very long time if they're maintained properly and not dry-cleaned after every wear. But the same can't be said for a black shirt.

Knit garments suffer multiple threats. Those that have been snagged can often be rethreaded or re-yarned and don't have to be thrown out, but if they have a huge hole then it may be time to move on, especially if it's in the middle of a pattern that would need to be rewoven. The same applies to pleated skirts—if you wash them and the pleats come out, it's almost impossible to find someone to put them back in.

Fuzz balls on sweaters are altogether more treatable. These are inevitable regardless of a garment's quality and material, be it cashmere or cotton, but they can be removed if you know how to attack them. There's the Remington Fuzz-Away Fabric Shaver, as well as the sweater-customized pumice stones, that are both wonderful for scraping off the balls. However, once the fabric starts to wear out in those areas where you get the fuzz balls, or when the fuzz is immovable, it's again time to bid your garment good-bye.

Always beware of perfume or heavy antiperspirants that can ruin a delicate yarn. Perfumes contain alcohol, and powder deodorants can stain. Therefore, clean your sweaters before storing with cedar—moths love perfume and sweat, and they'll feed off your garments all summer. What's more, it is very hard to get sweaters back into shape once the shape has been lost, and that's why the label often states that they must be hand washed, with no spin cycle. Sometimes you can over-wash garments too, so you have to find the right balance and determine which things must be laundered more often than others.

Yellow perspiration or deodorant stains are often impossible to remove, especially on white garments. There are only so many times you can take white clothes to the cleaners. That's why it's often wiser to have them laundered and pressed rather than dry-cleaned, because dry-cleaning chemicals—especially the cheaper ones—can turn whites yellow. And white garments also have a dull finish if they've been over–dry-cleaned.

Here are some general cleaning tips.

✦ Lingerie

This type of clothing must be washed in a lingerie bag. There's no other way of protecting it. Even on its gentlest setting, a machine can do so much damage. Lingerie will unravel and disintegrate before your very eyes, regardless of whether it's a cheap five-and-dime piece or a Calvin Klein.

✦ Cashmere Sweaters

It's sometimes better to hand wash than dry-clean. You can put a cashmere sweater in the machine on the gentle cycle, but if the garment has more than one color, the dry cleaner is a must—the colors may not all be colorfast.

✦ Fragile Garments

I often use baby shampoo on my celebrity clients' clothes, or even Ivory liquid dishwashing soap. You can never be *too* gentle.

✦ Silks

Silks are one of the most difficult fabrics to deal with because of their poor dye retention. Dry-clean them after every wear to preserve their color.

✦ Leather

Wet leather needs to dry naturally; otherwise it will waffle and harden. Just see what happens when boots, bags, jackets, and skirts are blow-dried or placed in front of the fire. Ignore my advice and you'll be sure to send that cow out to pasture.

STAIN SOLUTIONS

While it's always worth paying for a professional's expertise, emergencies (not least when traveling) sometimes force us to take stain removal into our own hands. Here are some DIY problem solvers.

Lipstick: Loosen the stain with a nonflammable dry-cleaning solvent, rubbing in the detergent until the stain's outline is gone, and then wash in the hottest water.

Grease: Sponge the spot with a mixture comprising 1 tablespoon salt and 4 tablespoons rubbing alcohol. Wash in the hottest water that is safe for the fabric, and if the spot remains, use a dry-cleaning solvent and rewash.

Red wine: If the stain is still wet, apply club soda, cover the patch with salt, and then leave it for a few hours. The crystals will absorb the red pigment. Otherwise, resort to a stain remover such as Shout, Spot Shot, or Wine Away.

Deodorant: If you need to get it off quick, drugstores sell marvelous deodorant sponges that don't destroy the garment. If you have time to wait around, sponge the problem area with white vinegar.

Ink: Pour denatured alcohol through the stain, rub in petroleum jelly, sponge with a nonflammable dry-cleaning solvent, and wash with a detergent and a bleach that is safe for the fabric. This is a labor of love, but at least it'll make the mark disappear (and make you forever more watchful of pens).

It's so fabulous to have a properly organized wardrobe that simplifies your life, helps you to make the right fashion choices, and ensures that your clothes don't have the shelf life of full-fat milk. You'll soon realize that it's definitely worth the start-up effort and then the routine maintenance. After all, given what you've learned so far by reading this book, there's little doubt that you'll soon be storing more and more clothing—the *right* clothing!

YOUR TRAVELING "CLOSET"

Packing is a drag when you don't know exactly what you'll need for your trip. Chances are you don't have a personal assistant to pack for you, and you're more likely to fly coach on a commercial carrier than in luxury on a private jet, so space is limited. Here are some tips on what to pack for everything from a weekend jaunt with friends to a fortnight's trip to Europe that will help you look stylish every step of the way.

As a general rule, pack things that can serve you in different ways—for instance, the black skirt worn with a blazer for a business meeting can be remixed at night with a sequined top. A sports jacket is always handy because it can be worn more formal, or casually with jeans and pumps. The ability to remix aptly minimizes the number of garments you need to take with you, a godsend for anyone toting luggage.

Travel with clothes that don't easily wrinkle, such as jersey knits. It's not a good idea to take a linen suit if you won't have the time to press it out. Accordingly, when packing to avoid wrinkles, turn your jackets inside out, and zip and button all your garments before folding them to cut down on the creases and maximize space. Also, always remember to pack your cosmetics in your carry-on, because there's nothing worse than finding leaked lotions or oils all over your garments. That can be a disaster big enough to make you wish you'd lost your luggage.

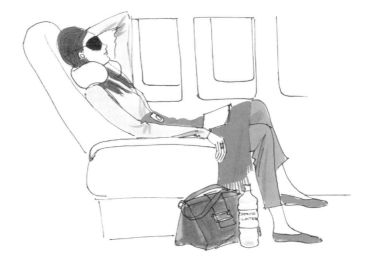

ITEMS YOU CAN'T LIVE WITHOUT ON A LONG JOURNEY EVEN AS YOU SIT IN COACH An ultrachic container for your carry-on pet; a bottle of Evian Mister for some much-needed hydration; some British tabloids to keep you occupied when the in-flight entertainment's a bore; a neck pillow that can also come in handy for your tired face and sore butt; eye cream to keep you looking fresh; sanitary hand wipes to keep you feeling clean; a sleep mask to help you relax; an iPod to help you chill out; and loose-fitting clothes and cashmere socks to keep you comfy and cozy.

The days of going to the airport in glamorous dresses or tight-fitting leather pants with a corseted top are over. Today, traveling in style means wearing loose clothes made out of luxury fabrics that are soft against your skin, don't cut off your circulation, and are easy to slip on and off. For some, it's all about the spaghetti-strap dress, jersey-knit pieces, and lingerie-tops-turned-outfits (sexy slips or lace camisoles); simple, one-piece outfits that won't wrinkle. I like to refer to this strategy as Marilyn Monroe Leisure Packing.

CURES FOR JET LAG Try to be rested, relaxed, and stress-free as you board the plane; drink lots of water during the flight to combat dehydration; and alternate in-flight rest with some walks up and down the aisle. Then, as soon as you arrive, book a massage so you'll feel rejuvenated and refreshed, and drink plenty of freshly squeezed juice to boost your energy. If that doesn't put you in vacation mode, go shopping!

CHAPTER TEN

THE MAN IN YOUR LIFE

BY NOW

I hope you're feeling like the next Jennifer Lopez. Nevertheless, wouldn't you like your husband or boyfriend to add a little star power to his own style?

It's great if your guy's appearance can actually complement yours, because there's nothing worse than seeing a woman totally decked out while her man stands nearby in sloppy clothes and a dirty pair of sneakers. So let's discuss how you can meet halfway before going out together for a night on the town. It doesn't mean matching Bobbsey Twins outfits, but at least go for subtle accents that will comple-ment one another, picking up on tones and perhaps even motifs in both of your outfits. You're each in your own space, but there's something that cosmically works together—it's more about the matching of personalities than it is about the matching of garments.

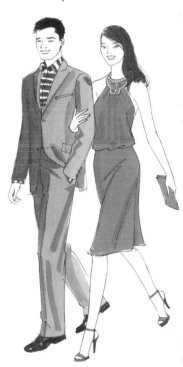

After all, even if your guy prefers the rocker look, there are numerous things he can do to complement your neatness without feeling that he's compromising his own grunginess. He can be grungy *and* neat, perhaps wearing a distressed jean that fits a little better, along with tops that match this style but don't make him look unkempt. Fit for a man is so important, especially with regard to suits and shirts—a baggy neck on a button-down shirt is unacceptable, and so are overlong sleeves on a smart blazer, boxy shoulders, or the hump that falls right in the middle of his back. Those little details can really make or break a guy's outfit.

It is not only a girl's place to get fussed over. A man should look just as well maintained, because this says a lot about his character. Most men will look at a woman if she's wearing a skirt that falls just below her butt or if she's showing extra cleavage and automatically think, "Oh, she's loose." Well, women also size up a man by gauging what he wears. Again, it's about the little details that serve as the finishing touch in terms of the overall look. This often amounts to good clothes that fit great, along with accessories that, while more understated than a woman's, are still classy. Indeed, a man can add class to his look by simply putting on a beautiful watch, wearing a terrific set of cuff links, or having his tie knotted to perfection. These are the things that really put my male clients over the top.

Make your man feel special. Okay, so he might not be as attached to his wardrobe as you are, but having his initials monogrammed onto his shirt cuffs is the kind of personal touch that will give him a sense of really owning his garments. At the same time, if he's the type who lives in a beat-up old sports jacket the same way that he's lived in a worn-out old leather chair throughout his bachelor existence, you have to tell him that it's time to update his look.

A man finds dressing complicated only when he hasn't yet defined his style. And when he does, it makes life so much easier. It's all down to who he is and, like you, the where, the when, and the why; where is he wearing the clothes, when is he wearing them, and why? If he's a corporate guy, his work wardrobe is pretty much laid out, with perhaps jeans, chinos, and some sports jackets fitting the bill for leisure. On the other hand, if he's a little more unconventional, the sky's the limit. Either way, it's easier for a man to define his style than it is for a woman to define hers, even though certain other considerations are strikingly similar.

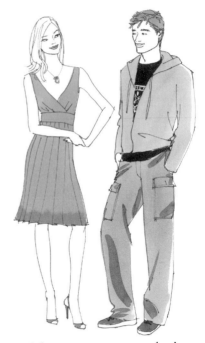

Just like you, he's going to need some key essentials. And it doesn't matter whether his style is Sean "Puffy" Combs, Ben Affleck, Jay-Z, or Jack Black. If he does sweatshirts and jeans the right way, he's going to look as hot as if he were wearing a Ralph Lauren suit. Of course, most guys don't enjoy shopping, so if you want to see a change, you'll probably have to do plenty of the legwork for him. This might mean a lot of store returns until you get it right, but he'll be relieved to have you take the job off his hands (even if he doesn't say so), and he'll appreciate your interest in upping his style when he gets compliments from everyone he knows. Believe me, girl, it's worth the effort . . . for *you* as well as for him!

WARDROBE ESSENTIALS FOR MEN

For men, the same general rules apply in terms of matching garments to body shape and size. For instance, guys who are heavy up top look really great in V-neck sweaters, but they should steer clear of turtlenecks, especially if they're short in the neck region. A double-breasted suit that's not fitted properly can create a bad look for heavy-chested men. Two- and three-button jackets look really great on guys who have a long torso, whereas average-shaped men look really sharp in one-button jackets.

Guys are often in denial about their body type. When getting fitted for a suit, there's nothing worse than the man who thinks he's a long when in reality he's a regular or a short. That can result in the jacket that comes to the knee—not a pretty sight. He's not supposed to be wearing a car coat as the top half of a suit. And neither should it look like a bolero jacket.

Let's get down to basics.

✦ The Black Suit

This versatile must-have is so important for both special and somber occasions, and it can be translated into any look. For instance, if your guy's style is a little more rocker, he can take the suit apart and pair the jacket with jeans and a T-shirt, or if he's a little more preppy, pair the jacket with khaki trousers, a cardigan sweater, and a gingham shirt. Whatever the scenario, he'll turn to this suit again and again. And he should also take note of the jacket's lining. Its color can be matched or contrasted with certain tops for added flair. However, unless he's a security guard at a high-end retail store, a black suit, black shirt, and black satin tie during the day are completely unacceptable.

✦ *If a guy has really broad shoulders, a peak lapel would be the first thing that I'd consider to make him look even broader. Then again, if he's going to a black-tie affair, where he needs something that's a little more extravagant, the peak lapel would provide the necessary drama, but he could also go for a notch lapel with a beautiful satin finish to contrast with a matte fabric on the body, and then add a tiepin to make him feel complete.*

✦ The Pinstripe or Herringbone Suit

In many cases more of a fashion piece than a necessity, this suit is nevertheless vital for the corporate businessman who wants to wear something that is both slimming and powerful in the boardroom. It can be navy, gray, chocolate, or black-and-white, although the navy blue will translate best from day to night. The point is, when in doubt, a man should wear a suit. It's smart and seasonless, and I guarantee it will announce his presence in any room.

✦ The Tuxedo

This always has a time and a place. And since it is classic and never goes out of season, there's no need to get this year's tuxedo. Instead, if money's an issue, it can be purchased at a Filene's Basement and numerous discount stores, or it can always be rented. Recently introduced accessories can also update the classic tux, such as a tiepin or a male brooch that is attached to the lapel—not something feminine and floral, but one that is, for example, feather- or sword-shaped—and also a silk scarf, placed on the inside of the lapel instead of the outside.

✦ The Sports Jacket

Regardless of texture, whether it's tweed, cotton, or nylon, depending on the season, the casual jacket is a staple that helps a man blend into countless environments. Styles include the car coat, the jean jacket, and the track jacket.

✦ The Overcoat

Vital for cold weather, if smart enough this can convey a definite power look while working for both dressy and casual occasions.

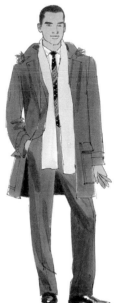

✦ The Parka

This warm knee- or thigh-length jacket with fur-lined hood is perfect for the fall. However, leave the waist-length parka off of your business suit. It's much more metropolitan to wear a three-quarter-length snorkel parka over a suit as you're tracking through the concrete jungle.

✦ The Button-Down Shirt

The smart button-down with a tab collar can be worn with or without a tie for different looks. However, it looks best with medium-width ties; the more casual, very American button-down is to be worn with a sports jacket. Incidentally, here's some advice concerning other types of collar.

The spread collar: The most dashing and confident, this looks great with a medium-to-wide tie knot; either a double-Windsor or four-in-hand.

The semi-spread collar: Flattering and forgiving, this is the everyman collar.

The long-pointed collar: Ideal under V-neck and crewneck sweaters as well as three-button suits, this works great with tie bars and skinny knots.

✦ The French-Cuff Shirt

Boasting a sleeve that is folded back and fastened with a cuff link, this is for more of a business or formal occasion, working great for both daytime and evening. Still, don't let your man feel pressured into wearing traditional business cuff links and a power tie, because depending on the environment he can also go with an open collar (lying *inside* the sports jacket lapel) and more creative links, be they wood, magnetized, or Lalique crystal. Just remember that, regardless of the cuff, he should always ensure that it fits correctly and shows when he's wearing a tailored suit.

The French cuff is, of course, the dressiest of the bunch. Here are some other available cuffs:

The single-button: This standard cuff should always reach to the hinge of the wrist.

The two-button barrel: for the guy who works well with an Italian-made suit but wants a shirt with British flair.

The convertible: Adjustable buttons allow for either narrow or wide cuffs; great for the guy who wears an oversize watch.

✦ THE POLO SHIRT
This can either be mixed with a sports jacket or worn casually on weekends, looking really good under a zip-front track jacket or sweater.

✦ THE V-NECK SWEATER
This is great for layering, by itself, or with a button-down shirt, depending on how extreme a guy's style is. Just remember that the button-down shirt's collar should be on the inside, never on the outside, unless he's trying to revive the look of some seventies disco outfit.

✦ THE CREWNECK SWEATER
Again, this is adaptable, but it's important to first stick to the solid colors—the reliable blues, grays, blacks—before adding accent colors. The ones that work best with his skin tone will serve as the fashion colors, be they yellow, powder blue, or even pink.

✦ THE CARDIGAN SWEATER
Essential for the more preppy guy or one who wants a smarter appearance. It lies great under a jacket and is a fabulous way of introducing color while playing down a look that is really serious.

✦ THE SMART-CASUAL TROUSERS
If pleats are the thing—and they are often the best choice for the more full-figured man—then one or two pleats are much smoother and cleaner than triple pleats, which will pucker too much with a protruding stomach. On the other hand, a guy with a medium-to-lean stomach might be better suited to wearing flat-front trousers. This European-inspired mod cut is for the man who wants a lean and clean finish. The smart-casual trouser works well with polos, T-shirts, and casual button-downs, and it should feel as comfortable as your favorite pair of jeans.

✦ The Jeans, Chinos, and Corduroys

All three are multipurpose essentials for casual evenings and weekends, with the cords replacing the chinos in the fall. No matter what a man wears up top, he cannot go wrong with these bottom basics. Dark-wash jeans are ideal, but the fit is down to personal preference, be it a baggier cut, a 501, a tapered leg, or a boot cut. Still, the guy who is barrel-shaped would be well advised to stay away from a taper-cut tight jean and go for more of a boot cut.

✦ The Plaid or Herringbone Pants

For the guy who is a little more on the edgy side, these can be matched with sports jackets to add some spice to his life. And if the vibe is right, he shouldn't be afraid to pair a tux jacket with his plaid or herringbone pants, keeping the shirt solid, of course. This will be a surefire conversation piece.

✦ The Dress Belts and Casual Belts

There should be several of these, including one in chocolate and one in black, each with gold and/or silver buckles. If there's a need or desire to be economical, reversible belts are a great option. And there can also be the rope sports/weekend belt; something a little more sporty to be worn with casual pants and jeans. Coordinating a belt with shoes is fine, but not a necessity, for a sporty look that allows your man to be more playful and introduce bright colors that don't match regular footwear. Just make sure he doesn't wear belts that are too narrow or too wide for his belt loops—this may sound obvious, but I've seen it all. Belts should be the finishing touch.

✦ Underwear

Tight briefs, loose boxers, or the in-between boxer briefs—this is such a personal choice. Some men prefer no underwear at all. However, even with underpants there are some obvious no-no's, like wearing yellow smiley-face boxers under cream trousers . . . unless that's the kind of statement your guy wishes to make. At the same time, when it comes to the top half of the body, it would be wise to have V-neck and crewneck T-shirts, as well as tank tops, to provide a little coverage under a sheer shirt or to inconspicuously keep itchy knits off the skin while adding a layer of warmth and preventing sweat marks.

✦ Swimsuits

The briefs aren't as popular as they used to be, although a lot of Europeans still wear them, so the boxer and Bermuda swimming trunks are usually the way to go, because they're flattering on a wide variety of body types.

✦ Must-Have Socks

It's so important to have good socks that are not going to ball up or fall apart after the first wash. This doesn't mean they have to be 100 percent cashmere— some blends last really well—but guys can certainly have a lot of fun in terms of the textures, colors, and patterns. They can coordinate them with their shirts or their ties or even the linings of their suits, and in that way use the socks to exhibit a little personality, not least when they sit down and cross their legs. If being worn with a black or brown suit, for example, the socks should provide something very rich as opposed to an ashy gray contrast; black on black, or a great color for the eyes to pick up, such as red or mint green. Just remember, the socks should always match the trousers or, if the guy is a bit more on the adventurous side, his shirt. Then again, the man who wears bright red socks with a dark suit is James Bond all the way: adventurous and thrilling.

✦ Must-Have Shoes

Black dress shoes are vital, as are chocolate or natural driving loafers and/or suede shoes for laid-back evenings, casual Fridays, and weekends. Then there are the tennis sneakers, whether they're for fashion or athletic purposes; the sandals for vacations; and the dress boots, be they lace-up or slip-on, that work well day to evening. Shoes should be rotated according to season, and also for durability, so make sure you always have more than one option. Go for a sleeker, cleaner, less trendy shoe if you're looking to economize, and stay away from a square toe at all costs, as this is an obvious trend that will automatically date you.

ACCESSORIZING FOR MEN

A man can really find things to define his personal style. In fact, there are nearly as many options for him as there are for you, so let's work our way again from top to bottom.

✦ HATS

A hat is like a pair of glasses—the shape of the face plays a big part in terms of what works best, and so does personal style.

Fedoras and rain hats are always popular, while wool hats, trucker hats, and thermal skullcaps are fashionable among rockers and skate-boarders. Then again, newsboy hats can play a look up or down, making a tracksuit look like a business suit and a business suit look like a track-suit. The same applies to baseball caps, which can be worn regular or back-to-front depending on what kind of day your man is having; the peak at the front if he wants a practical way of shading his eyes from the sun, and the other way around if he's feeling a bit more rambunctious.

Of course, thinning hair is a much more widespread concern for men than it is for women, and hats can serve as a safe and reliable option for those who aren't too comfortable about exposing their baldness or who need to conceal an ill-shaped dome. Desperately holding on to what hair there is can make them look older—the ponytail and comb-over only emphasize what's missing—so they're best advised to toughen up, face reality, and adopt trendy headwear when they want to add some style up top.

✦ EYEWEAR

This offers the same dramatic attribute to men as it does to women; that air of mystery: "Who's *that* guy?" He automatically appears more sensational and sexy when he puts on a pair of glasses, and they don't have to be shades, either. For some guys, putting on the right pair of specs makes them look smarter, older (if they're baby-faced), and more chic and sophisticated—just look at Spike Lee. He's iconic for his glasses.

✦ Neckwear

Ties

These can clearly express a man's unique personality and attitude, presenting endless options and possibilities. They are like earrings, coordinating with the color combinations that guys put together. Still, it's always good to have a solid black tie and white tie in terms of the basics (along with at least one bow tie in waiting for a black-tie event). Indeed, the young and hip even go for things that are a little more adventurous, merging polka-dot ties with gingham shirts that look great underneath the pinstripes, or going with stripe on stripe.

The days of monochromatic shirt-tie combos have passed, and men can now enjoy adding personal style to their lives with something more punchy—reverse pencil stripes, mini checks, windowpane, gingham, and awning stripes can all serve as the starting point for jazzing up a pinstripe or khaki suit that is thirsty for color. The tie is an open field, and when mixing patterns with any type of shirt it's sure to be a conversation piece. Then again, a tie that has a rich, solid color can also be very powerful, so a man should never feel obliged to match more than he's comfortable with. Just ensure that the tip of his tie reaches to the top of the waistband. There's nothing worse than a tie that reaches to the bellybutton or past the zipper.

As for choosing a knot, a tie that has a little more weight lends itself best to the fuller knot—a single or double Windsor—whereas less weight is preferable to achieve a smaller, more retro, 1960s kind of knot. I remember when Jay-Z first started wearing suits, for instance; his knots were kind of loose, had no definition, and didn't convey his powerful personality, so I introduced him to the double Windsor, and through his example it became really popular among the masses. This is a well-defined knot that is very cocky and very strong, whereas the smaller retro knot is much more sleek and slick.

Tie Bars and Tie Clips
These are very popular and they're great accessories, almost like necklaces, helping to create a finished look. A man doesn't *need* a tie bar, but it really adds that extra strong element.

Scarves
These can range from an ascot to a silk scarf that is just tucked inside the shirt and lies nicely for more of an Italian/French kind of look, or worn on top of a jacket for the James Bond or mafioso effect. Then there are the cashmere scarves that can be thrown over a top and jacket—these can even play beautifully with jogging suits, baseball hats, and sneakers when guys are traveling, adding a sense of richness to give that over-the-top look.

✦ SUSPENDERS
These are functional and they never go out of style, but again they come down to personal preference. Guys who like them should go for the ones that button inside the waistband, not those with metal clips. And they shouldn't be worn with a belt, because braces are already there to hold the pants up. Yet another expression of a man's personality, and a very retro one at that. Just stay away from overly commercial or gimmicky patterns, as is the case with ties.

✦ JEWELRY
This should never be overdone, but should be understated, subtle, and sophisticated. Sure, it may be fashionable for guys onstage to wear loads of chains and diamond rings, but such exaggeration really won't work for the traditional man who's looking to incorporate superstar quality into his life. He can have a diamond cuff link, but it shouldn't be the size

of his thumb, and the same with rings—there's nothing wrong with having a pinky ring, but it should definitely be more on the subtle side rather than look like it goes with a cane and whiskey sipping cup. A simple chain is very sexy on a man, and some are even getting into pearls right now, although that's a very extreme look. Otherwise, a regular watch and dress watch are obligatory. A watch is the strongest bracelet a man can have, and it becomes just as much a conversation piece for him as shoes are for a woman.

✦ Man Purses

There is the messenger bag for the trendy younger man on the go, the briefcase for the office type, the envelope clutch for entrepreneurial essentials, the doctor's bag that serves as a mobile office, the weekend duffel bag for leisure, and the knapsack for the hands-free backpacker. However, the choices are minimal compared to women's pocketbooks. Many men have one or two bags and they fall in love with them forever. Luckily for guys, a little worn-in character is considered ideal.

DRESSING HIS AGE

Men, too, should dress according to their years. This is so important, as evidenced by the ridiculous sight of a middle-aged man wearing tons of chains, a motorcycle jacket, a tank top, and a distressed, hole-filled pair of baggy jeans. That's a nightmare. A gentleman should look like a gentleman and dress accordingly. I don't expect to see a forty-year-old guy in a basketball jersey and a pair of trousers, and I also don't want to see him looking like he's way past his sell-by date. It's basically nice to see him looking a little bit hip and trendy without trying to give the impression that he's just about old enough to drink. And with that in mind, he should look to wear the things that carry over to any age group, such as polo shirts.

Since there's a good chance that your guy's natural instinct is to be in control—at least of his own life—it may be easier said than done to get him to follow your style advice. However, if you're subtle, you can succeed. Try laying out his clothes to save him the effort, and slip in a few new ones that you want to see him in, such as a new sweater or some cool underwear. Just pick up whatever you want to change about him, and also buy a few men's magazines and leave them in the bathroom to help ignite his appetite for the world of fashion. Make him aware of style and introduce him to the concept of taking an active role in his look.

Like you, your mate needs to find things that not only work visually but that he also feels comfortable wearing, both mentally and physically. He may know quicker than you when a garment that he puts on feels good, yet there *are* ways for you to make a change. You just have to remember that most things your guy owns are very personal to him and that he likes to retain control, so be careful and diplomatic in terms of your approach. And after all that, if he still won't fall into line, don't feel obliged to kick him to the curb. Just take him to his favorite retail store, seeking out assistance from a salesman/personal shopper, and hopefully your efforts to improve his overall look and attitude toward style will eventually persuade him to complement your own. *That's love.*

MALE STYLE ICONS TO LEARN FROM

CARY GRANT This man was so suave, slick, and neat, tailored to perfection without ever being overdone, and he paid such great attention to detail. Classy and classic, he is a timeless reference for generations of men the world over.

SIDNEY POITIER Absolute genius. He wears black tie as naturally as his birthday suit. The same applies to Harry Belafonte.

JAY-Z Here's a guy who has gone from being a hip-hop artist to a music industry executive, and his transformation was so natural and organic that it became his second skin. From a denim suit to jeans and a button-down shirt and then to a button-down shirt and a pair of trousers, he slowly and subtly evolved into a music-biz fashion icon, where people now recognize him for his style.

SEAN "PUFFY" COMBS He has a very bold way of cultivating fashion. The way he wears things is like nobody else, doing it in a very big way, and most of the time very inspired by the 1940s and that mobster/bad boy kind of look. The fact that he pulls it off so well is not due to a gangster attitude, but his swagger and his confidence. The way he puts things on is just killer—the eclectic combination of diverse elements such as the overcoat with the tux jacket, jeans, combat boots, and glasses conveys the aura of a superstar. There's a certain kind of confidence that men need to own and command their image, and "Puffy" has that in abundance.

JUDE LAW More traditional, he nevertheless goes for modern touches like little scarves and puts himself together really well.

DAVID BECKHAM He has embraced the whole metrosexual persona, illustrating how even a guy can feel totally at ease in women's shirts and his wife's underwear, and look really cool and manly in kilts, ruffled shirts, and any number of dandified items.

AFTERWORD

FINDING

yourself in terms of your clothes and your look is an intricate journey, and while we have covered a lot of ground in this book, we've still only skimmed the surface.

Achieving your goals rarely happens in a flash. There are endless possibilities when it comes to cultivating who you are by way of your style. And like your personality, inspiration continues to evolve, so keep your eyes and your mind open, and embrace change. After all, now that you have the foundation, you can build on top of it, time and again.

My hope is that *Effortless Style* has provided you with the confidence to enrich your life through wardrobe. You now understand the strength that you can derive from changing your appearance so that your outer look gives expression to your inner self. *Who am I? Who do I want to be? Who have I become?* If you can answer these questions, then I've done my job. In the end, it's all about discovering and celebrating the truly unique and fabulous person that you can be.

Celebrity fashion stylist/designer JUNE AMBROSE has appeared on national shows including *The Oprah Winfrey Show*, *The View*, *Live with Regis and Kelly*, and *Extreme Makeover*, and on VH1 and MTV. She owns the full-service styling firm The Modé Squad, Inc. in New York City.

RICHARD BUSKIN is the *New York Times* bestselling author of more than a dozen books on subjects ranging from Marilyn Monroe and Princess Diana to The Beatles and Sheryl Crow.

AIMEE LEVY's illustrations appear in *Allure*, *Cosmopolitan*, *Marie Claire Italia*, *Brides UK*, *Condé Nast Traveller*, and numerous other magazines. She has created illustrations for cosmetic companies, including L'Oréal, Coty, and Merle Norman, and she has illustrated many book covers. A native New Yorker, she now lives in Santa Monica, California.